Cultural Competency in Psychological Assessment

ABCT Clinical Practice Series

Series Editor

Jordana Muroff, PhD, LICSW, Associate Professor and Chair, Clinical Practice Department, Boston University School of Social Work

Associate Editors

Anu Asnaani, PhD, Assistant Professor, Department of Psychology, University of Utah

Lara J. Farrell, PhD, Associate Professor, School of Applied Psychology, Griffith University and Menzies Health Institute of Queensland, Australia

Matthew A. Jarrett, PhD, Associate Professor, Department of Psychology, University of Alabama

Titles in the Series

Applications of the Unified Protocol for Transdiagnostic Treatment of Emotional Disorders
Edited by David H. Barlow and Todd Farchione

Helping Families of Youth with School Attendance Problems
Christopher A. Kearney

Addressing Parental Accommodation When Treating Anxiety in Children
Eli R. Lebowitz

Exposure Therapy for Eating Disorders
Carolyn Black Becker, Nicholas R. Farrell, and Glenn Waller

Exposure Therapy for Child and Adolescent Anxiety and OCD
Stephen P. H. Whiteside, Thomas H. Ollendick, and Bridget K. Biggs

Managing Microaggressions
Monnica T. Williams

A Clinician's Guide to Disclosures of Sexual Assault
Amie R. Newins and Laura C. Wilson

Applications of the Unified Protocols for Transdiagnostic Treatment of Emotional Disorders in Children and Adolescents
Jill Ehrenreich-May and Sarah M. Kennedy

Cultural Competency in Psychological Assessment

Working Effectively with Latinx Populations

ALFONSO MERCADO

AND

AMANDA VENTA

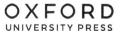

OXFORD
UNIVERSITY PRESS

Oxford University Press is a department of the University of Oxford. It furthers
the University's objective of excellence in research, scholarship, and education
by publishing worldwide. Oxford is a registered trade mark of Oxford University
Press in the UK and certain other countries.

Published in the United States of America by Oxford University Press
198 Madison Avenue, New York, NY 10016, United States of America.

Library of Congress Cataloging-in-Publication Data
Names: Mercado, Alfonso (Psychologist), author. | Venta, Amanda, 1987– author.
Title: Cultural competency in psychological assessment : working effectively with
Latinx populations / Alfonso Mercado, Amanda Venta.
Description: New York, NY : Oxford University Press, [2023] |
Series: ABCT clinical practice series | Includes bibliographical references and index.
Identifiers: LCCN 2022030853 (print) | LCCN 2022030854 (ebook) |
ISBN 9780190065225 (paperback) | ISBN 9780190065249 (epub) |
ISBN 9780190065256 (ebook)
Subjects: LCSH: Hispanic Americans—Mental health services—United States. |
Hispanic Americans—Mental health—United States. | Latin Americans—Mental health
services—United States. | Latin Americans—Mental health—United States. | Immigrants—
Mental health services—United States. | Immigrants—Mental health—United States. |
Psychiatry, Transcultural—United States. | Cross-cultural counseling—United States. |
Intercultural communication—United States.
Classification: LCC RC451.5.H57 M47 2023 (print) | LCC RC451.5.H57 (ebook) |
DDC 362.196/89068073—dc23/eng/20220716
LC record available at https://lccn.loc.gov/2022030853
LC ebook record available at https://lccn.loc.gov/2022030854

DOI: 10.1093/med-psych/9780190065225.001.0001

9 8 7 6 5 4 3 2 1

Printed by Lakeside Book Company, United States of America

CONTENTS

FOREWORD

Mental health clinicians are ardently committed to collaborating with their clients and helping them while recognizing the importance of implementing evidence-based treatments toward achieving this goal. Over the past several years, the field of mental healthcare has seen tremendous advances in our understanding of mental health challenges and their underlying mechanisms as well as the proliferation and refinement of scientifically informed treatment approaches. Coinciding with these advances is a heightened focus on accountability in clinical practice. Clinicians are expected to apply evidence-based approaches and do so effectively, efficiently, and in a patient-centered, individualized way. Delivery of evidence-based approaches can be challenging for a multitude of reasons, including but not limited to structural barriers to care and oppressive factors, responsiveness to a client's cultural and contextual factors, and the complexity of mental health challenges (e.g., comorbidity).

This series, which represents a collaborative effort between the Association for Behavioral and Cognitive Therapies (ABCT) and Oxford University Press, is intended to serve as an easy-to-use, highly practical collection of resources for clinicians and trainees. The *ABCT Clinical Practice Series* is designed to help clinicians effectively master and implement evidence-based treatment approaches. In practical terms, the series represents the "brass tacks" of implementation, including basic how-to guidance and advice on troubleshooting common issues in clinical practice and application. As such, the series is best viewed as a complement to other series on evidence-based protocols such as the *Treatments That Work*™ series and the *Programs That Work*™ series. These represent seminal bridges between research and practice and have been instrumental in the dissemination of empirically supported intervention protocols and programs. The *ABCT Clinical Practice Series*, rather than focusing on specific diagnoses and their treatment, targets the practical application of therapeutic and assessment approaches. In other words, the emphasis is on the *how-to* aspects of mental health delivery.

It is my hope that clinicians and trainees find these books useful in refining their clinical skills because enhanced comfort as well as competence in delivery of evidence-based approaches should ultimately lead to improved client outcomes.

Given the emphasis on application in this Series, there is relatively less emphasis on review of the underlying research base. Readers who wish to delve more deeply into the theoretical or empirical basis supporting specific approaches are encouraged to go to the original source publications cited in each chapter. When relevant, suggestions for further reading are provided.

In this book, Drs. Alfonso Mercado and Amanda Venta focus on culturally sensitive assessment practices with Latinx persons. The Latinx population has experienced fast growth and is highly diverse in terms of immigration status, being born in the United States or in other countries of origin, cultural variation, skin color, language preference, acculturation, and intersecting identities. Access to linguistically and culturally relevant services is crucial yet extremely limited. Assessment is an essential aspect of ethical mental health practice and has significant implications at the time it is conducted as well as in the future.

Drs. Mercado and Venta discuss the critical need and provide guidance for conducting assessment processes with Latinx persons that incorporate cultural competency and humility, Latinx cultural values, and cultural conceptualization. Additionally, specific mental health assessment tools are discussed regarding their strengths and limitations in their applications with Latinx populations, and helpful considerations for selection are provided. Outstanding insights and practical applications are offered regarding linguistic considerations, working with interpreters, dealing with prejudice and microaggressions, working with undocumented and immigrant clients including children, and recommendations for future research. Drs. Mercado and Venta's extensive experience collaborating with Latinx communities and their deep understanding of factors contextualizing the assessment of Latinx clients are shared in a clear, concise, comprehensive, and timely guide that is likely to inform clinical decision-making and enhance the practice of mental health trainees and clinicians with varying levels of experience and from numerous professional backgrounds.

—Jordana Muroff, PhD, LICSW
Series Editor

Introduction

We begin this volume by introducing what we hope is valuable context for the remainder of the text. After introducing ourselves, we provide background in a number of areas that contextualize later chapters. Specifically, we address diversity within Latinx populations, including the intersection of Latinx and immigrant identities. Several topics important in the Latinx mental health literature, like the Hispanic Health Paradox, the Immigrant Paradox, acculturation, and acculturative stress are introduced. The special case of unaccompanied immigrant minors, a section of the Latinx population that has grown rapidly in the United States over the past decade, is also described. We also present relevant ethical principles and codes of conduct relevant to working with Latinx persons and make our case of the importance of culturally sensitive assessment practices.

CLINICAL EXPERIENCE OF AUTHORS

Dr. Alfonso Mercado, originally from Los Angeles, California, is Associate Professor in the Department of Psychological Science and Department of Psychiatry in the School of Medicine at the University of Texas-Rio Grande Valley and a licensed psychologist. He is also a National Register Health Service psychologist and provides psychological services in an underserved community on the US–Mexico border. Dr. Mercado is also a visiting professor at the Universidad de Guadalajara in Jalisco, Mexico, and at the Universidad Central de Ecuador in Quito. His Multicultural Clinical lab focuses on Latinx mental health including immigration, personality, substance misuse, and multicultural interventions. He is President of the Texas Psychological Association and elected leader in the Committee on Rural Health at the American Psychological Association. Dr. Mercado has extensive clinical experience working with various culturally diverse groups. Since the influx of unaccompanied minors crossing the Rio Grande River of Texas in 2014, Dr. Mercado has provided psychological evaluations to children, adolescents, and families from Central America and many other regions. In 2018, he provided psychological services to children who experienced family separations. In addition to providing psychological evaluations to this population,

Dr. Mercado also conducts psychological evaluations for immigration purposes. Dr. Mercado led a task force at the National Latinx Psychological Association to develop the first professional guidelines for psychological evaluations used in immigration proceedings, which were published in 2022. Dr. Mercado is a first-generation American of Mexican heritage and a Spanish-English bilingual researcher, supervisor, and service provider.

Dr. Amanda Venta is Associate Professor of Psychology at the University of Houston. Her primary research interests are the development of psychopathology in youth and the protective effect of attachment security. Much of her clinical work has focused on the psychological functioning of recently immigrated youth and families from Central America, including providing psychological services for the Office of Refugee Resettlement since 2012. Dr. Venta has completed hundreds of psychodiagnostic evaluations of this type. Her research has also expanded to include a focus on immigrant youth and families, examining their mental health utilizing the perspectives of developmental psychopathology and attachment theory. Research projects in this vein include a longitudinal study of risk and protective factors for psychopathology in recently immigrated teens, a study of mental and physical health in mothers and children who have crossed the US–Mexico border within the last 24 hours (with Dr. Mercado), and an examination of immune function in the context of trauma among immigrant youth. Her research has received funding from the National Institute of Mental Health and, more recently, the National Institute of Minority Health and Health Disparities. Dr. Venta is a first-generation American of Cuban heritage and a Spanish-English bilingual researcher, supervisor, and service provider.

LATINX PERSONS IN THE UNITED STATES

Diversity in Latinx Groups

Latinx persons in the United States are a hugely diverse group. The Pew Research Center, in 2019, published the following key facts about US Hispanics that make this statement clear (Noe-Bustamante, 2019). Among the overall population of more than 58 million Latinx persons, they cite significant populations from 15 nations that differ widely from one another. More than 36 million Latinx persons in the United States self-report being from Mexico, a country in North America with a very different history and relationship with the United States than Spain (from which 810,000 US Latinx persons originate) or Argentina (from which 278,000 US Latinx persons originate). There is important diversity within these groups as well. For example, Cuban Americans tend to be older, with a median age of 40 reported, in contrast to Mexicans, who reported a mean age of only 27. Their level of education is widely different as well, with 55% of Venezuelans reporting at least a bachelor's degree, compared with 10% of Salvadorans or Guatemalans in the United States. As we will discuss in subsequent chapters of this book, Latinx persons in the United States are differentially affected by immigration-related variables. While 91% of Spaniards and 99% of Puerto Ricans are US citizens, only about half of Venezuelans, Guatemalans, and Hondurans are citizens. Indeed, most Spaniards in the United States were actually born in here (16% foreign-born), which is not true for Dominicans, Nicaraguans, Cubans, Salvadorans, Ecuadorians, Argentines, Guatemalans, Colombians, Hondurans, Peruvians, or Venezuelans who range between 54% and 74% foreign born. Latinx persons in the United States also vary tremendously in income and access to healthcare, with only 9% of Argentines living in poverty and 12% lacking health insurance, in contrast with 26% of Hondurans living in poverty and 35% lacking health insurance. Working effectively with Latinx persons means recognizing that Latinx people are diverse and that one Latinx client may be very different from another along the seven dimensions just discussed and many more that we haven't reviewed.

Most existing studies in psychology fail to represent the diversity among Latinx persons. Indeed, most research studies, as summarized by McLaughlin et al. (2007), fail to define their ethnic/racial group divisions accurately and rely on Black versus White divisions or Black versus White versus Latinx groups (Bird, 1996; McLaughlin et al., 2007). This approach has important limitations. First, many of these studies fail to recognize Latinx people at all, using only racial categories of White and Black to represent their samples. Alternatively, some studies conceptualize their samples as including participants from ethnic minority groups and those who do not belong in ethnic minority groups, pairing Black and Latinx participants together as though they are the same because they are both from groups that represent minority racial/ethnic groups in the United States. Second, these approaches to categorization ignore the fact that racial and ethnic categories are not mutually exclusive. For example, people can be Black and Hispanic and White and Hispanic. Indeed, all two-group comparison studies focused on racial makeup fail to reflect racial heterogeneity among Hispanics—of whom about 53% identify as White, 2.5% as Black, and the remainder (44.5%) as belonging to some other, or multiple, racial groups (Humes, Jones, & Ramirez, 2011). Third, even studies that look at race as one dimension (e.g., White, Black) and ethnicity as a separate dimension (e.g., Latinx, non-Latinx) frequently group all Latinx persons together, often due to limitations in sample size. Latinx people in the United States are from different cultures, countries, and even continents. Grouping them all together as Hispanics fails to recognize diversity within Latinx communities, including skin color. Finally, there are added complexities once one recognizes that, for example, the gender-based differences that have been well-documented in White Americans are likely present in Latinx persons as well and that, therefore, looking at Latinx people, even of one cultural group, as a homogeneous group is overlooking important diversity along other lines (e.g., gender; McLaughlin et al., 2007).

Another important dimension on which Latinx people in the United States differ is acculturation—a bidimensional process in which an individual will range from high to low on affiliation with their host (post-migration) culture and, on a separate axis, from high to low on affiliation with their culture of origin (Sam & Berry, 2010). There are many studies that show a relation between acculturation and important mental health variables that will be reviewed elsewhere in this book. In this section, though, it is important to recognize that Latinx persons in the United States (even those who are from the same country or culture and those who are of the same gender and socioeconomic status) will differ based on how much they identify with their culture of origin and how much they identify with their host culture. Individuals high in affiliation with their host culture and low in affiliation with their culture of origin, for instance, are described as "assimilated," whereas individuals high on both axes are referred to as "bicultural/integrated." Individuals low in both metrics are described as "marginalized," and individuals with high affiliation with their culture of origin only are referred to as "traditional/ separated." Overall, acculturation is conceptualized as a change in cultural identity, one that includes shifts in various cultural dimensions including typical practices, values, and identifications (Schwarz et al., 2009). Importantly, the process of acculturation is relevant across generations of immigrants, meaning that even US-born Latinx persons will range in their level of acculturation. Take, for example, two siblings in the same family of Cuban American immigrants. One of them was born in a Cuban American neighborhood in Miami and raised surrounded by extended family of Cuban origin. Another sibling, even though they had the same parents, socioeconomic status, and even gender, was raised in the Pacific Northwest after the family moved. That sibling would have spent less time surrounded by Cuban food, family, and cultural traditions—the siblings likely vary greatly on their acculturation, and mental health professionals would do a disservice in ignoring this variation. They may also have important differences in the extent to which they have experience perceived racism and discrimination—experiences that have been linked to negative mental health and academic outcomes in Latinx people (Smokowski & Bacallao, 2006; Suárez-Orozco, Rhodes, & Milburn, 2009)—as a factor of the dominant cultural group that surrounds them.

Recognizing acculturation as an important within-group difference among Latinx persons highlights a fifth way in which much of psychological research has failed to recognize diversity within US Latinx groups. Indeed, in ethnic group comparison studies, group designs rarely assess self-identified cultural group dominance and collapse all Latinx persons together into one group, ignoring important within-group diversity in acculturation by focusing on Latinx versus White or Latinx versus Black differences. This picture grows even more complex when recognizing that acculturation itself, if it is even included in a study, could be measured using different instruments, defined differently across studies, or even treated as though it is synonymous with acculturative stress—self-reported distress during the acculturation process (e.g., distress associated with speaking with an accent; Bulut & Gayman, 2015; Teruya & Bazargan-Hejazi, 2013).

Latinx Immigration in the United States

Not all Latinx people in the United States are immigrants, and it is a mistake to equate the terms *immigrant* and *Latinx*. Indeed, only 33% of Latinx persons in the United States were born outside of the country (Noe-Bustamante, 2019), and, among the top five countries of birth for immigrants in the United States, there are only two Latin American nations (i.e., Mexico and El Salvador, among China, India, and the Philippines; Radford, 2019). Furthermore, it is important that we do not stereotype the Latinx immigrant as a poor, undocumented, newcomer to the United States. Immigrants are actually a declining percentage of the US Latinx population (i.e., 40% in 2000 compared with 33% in 2017): 79% of US Latinx persons are US citizens, 78% have lived in the country for more than 10 years, and only 19% live in poverty (Noe-Bustamante, 2019). While recognizing the diversity within immigrant groups is essential, mental health professionals working with Latinx persons will inevitably serve immigrants in schools, clinics, hospitals, and prisons (Casas, 2017), making immigration an important topic within Latinx mental health more broadly. Indeed, the United States is home to approximately 40.4 million immigrants (US Census Bureau, 2011), of which one-third are from Mexico and 55% originate from Latin-America (US Census Bureau, 2011).

When a foreign-born person settles in the United States, they are defined as an immigrant. Immigrant status can vary widely, and we know that some groups of immigrants may access mental health resources more or less than others. Broadly, an immigrant status could include becoming a citizen, a lawful permanent resident, a refugee, an asylum seeker, or an undocumented immigrant (Bourke, 2014). An undocumented immigrant is someone who entered the United States without the proper legal authorization or entered with legal authorization but violated the terms of the visa status. While many people think of undocumented immigrants as those who cross the US–Mexico border under the cover of darkness, a report by the Center for Migration Studies of New York reveals that visa overstays are much more prevalent than we think—exceeding illegal border crossings every year between 2010 and 2017 (Warren, 2019). One current estimate of America's undocumented immigrant population is 11.7 million (Passel, Cohn, & Gonzalez-Barrera, 2013).

According to the United Nations High Commission on Refugees (UNHCR, 2012), a main difference between immigrants and refugees is that immigrants choose to move to the United States not because of a direct threat of persecution or death, as in the case of refugees, but mainly to improve their lives (e.g., financially, educationally, due to family reunion, or other reasons). Thus, a *refugee* is defined as a person fleeing natural disaster, armed conflict, or persecution based on race, religion, nationality, or political opinion (Bourke, 2014; United Nations General Assembly, 1951). An *asylum seeker* is someone who claims to be a refugee but has not yet had his or her case evaluated or accepted. To qualify for asylum in the United States, the applicant must demonstrate to US immigration officials that (1) he or she fears persecution; (2) the persecution would occur based on race, religion, nationality, political opinion, or social group; and (3) that the home country government is either involved in the persecution or unable to control it (Bourke, 2014). While media outlets have recently featured many families and children from Central America who are seeking asylum in the United States, it is important to see the whole picture: in 2015, the United States granted refugee status to 2,050 individuals from Latin America, 2,363 from Europe, 18,469 from

Asia, 22,472 from Africa, and 24,579 from South Asia (UNHCR, 2017). Given the large number of immigrants to the United States who are granted refugee status, and the even larger number who have similar experiences but either do not seek or are denied refugee status, it is important to recognize that immigrants to the United States differ in their reasons for migrating to the country. Some are escaping violence and poverty, motivating applications for asylum, whereas others receive sponsorship from an employer because they have specific skills or training needs in the United States, and still others are motivated to reunite with family members who have been living in the United States for a long time. These motivations for migration, just like immigration status once in the United States, are important factors representing the diversity of immigrants in the United States and must be considered in meeting their mental health needs. In the sections that follow we discuss the very specific case of unaccompanied immigrant minors, a rapidly growing demographic in the United States and one that has received a lot of media attention.

Unaccompanied Immigrant Minors

One unique immigrant population that mental health professionals may encounter in the clinical practice includes unaccompanied minors, which include children and teenagers seeking asylum from Central America. The past 5 years have seen a significant rise of migration in this form. Media outlets have widely broadcast images of children in ramshackle shelters at our southern border and children wrapped in aluminum blankets in temporary detention centers. In recent years, there have been unprecedented increases in youth migration to the United States from Central America—particularly El Salvador, Guatemala, and Honduras—where crime, death, and violence have reached record levels. This shift is recent, with Honduras reporting the highest homicide rate globally in 2011; 2013 marking the end of a truce between major gang powers in El Salvador; and crime victimization was cited as a major reason for Central American migration in 2014 (Hiskey et al., 2016). As the sociopolitical climate of Central America has changed, so, too, have patterns of Latinx immigration to the United States. Between 2015 and 2016 alone, there was a 131% increase in the number of children and families crossing the southwestern border of the United States reflecting large numbers of families seeking "humanitarian protection" (US Customs and Border Protection, Southwest Border Sectors, 2016). Dramatic increases in rates of crime, violence, and death in Central American have corresponded to increases in reports of trauma and posttraumatic symptoms among recent waves of Hispanic immigrants (US Conference on Catholic Bishops, 2015). This group of immigrants warrants the attention of psychologists due to its rapid growth in recent years as well as their particular vulnerability (Venta, 2019; Venta & Mercado, 2019).

The US Homeland Security Act of 2002 (Homeland Security, 2002) defined unaccompanied minors as children who have no lawful immigration status in the United States, have not reached 18 years of age, and have no legal guardian available in the United States. In 2010, there were 1 million children included in the estimated 11.1 million undocumented immigrants living in the United States (Passel & Cohn, 2012). In 2015, there were more than 32,000 apprehensions of children with at least one guardian and 28,000 apprehensions of unaccompanied children traveling across the US–Mexico border (Krogstad, 2016). During 2016 alone, almost 60,000 unaccompanied minors were taken into custody at the border (US Customs and Border Protection, 2016).

Once an unaccompanied minor is apprehended crossing the US–Mexico border, regardless of his or her potential future legal outcome (e.g., refugee, deportation, asylum), he or she is taken to a detention center for hours or days. Immigration officials then determine whether each migrant is younger than 18, is undocumented, and has potential guardians in the United States. If all these criteria are met, the child carries the legal term of "unaccompanied alien child" (USICS, n.d.). Officials gather data on each child's family background, identify potential security risks (e.g., gang affiliation), and make a preliminary recommendation for placement in the Unaccompanied Refugee Minors Program operated by the Office of Refugee Resettlement (ORR). Minors can be placed in a shelter facility, foster care, or group home; staff-secure or secure care facility; residential treatment center; or other special needs care facility based on their needs. Typically, placement decisions are made based on the following considerations: trafficking or safety concerns, special mental health or medical concerns, possibility of heightened vulnerability to sexual abuse, prior sexual abuse, sexual orientation, location of potential sponsor, sibling in ORR custody, legal representation needs, behavioral problems, criminal background, danger to self/community, escape risk, age, gender, length of stay, and location of apprehension (Office of Refugee Resettlement [ORR], 2015).

Understanding the legal process and what the unaccompanied children experience upon arrival to the United States is very important. As psychologists and mental health professionals, we have a duty to do no harm and assure we conduct psychological evaluations and facilitate mental health interventions in an ethical manner. It is imperative that clinicians conduct assessments that are culturally relevant, responsive, and informed by research. This book will touch on important components of the psychological evaluation process, including clinical interviewing and assessment via a cultural lens when working with immigrant groups and the Latinx population. One related health model used to better understand the Latinx and immigrant population is that of the *Hispanic Health Paradox*.

The Hispanic Health Paradox and the Immigrant Paradox

Any discussion on serving the mental health needs of Latinx persons in the United States must include some background on research that has shown that Latinx people in the United States are tremendously resilient. The *Hispanic Health Paradox* refers to an existing literature base showing that, despite exposure to many health risks like low socioeconomic status, limited access to healthcare and insurance, and reduced education and employment, Latinx persons in the United States generally report better health than non-Latinx Whites (Ruiz et al., 2016). This effect is even more pronounced among Latinx immigrants (i.e., foreign born; Singh, Rodriguez-Lainz, & Kogan, 2013), and a similar construct called the *Immigrant Paradox* suggests that first-generation immigrants are at a lower risk for a range of health problems and psychopathology than their native-born counterparts, despite sociological disadvantage (Acevedo-Garcia & Bates, 2008; Lui, 2015; MacDonald & Saunders, 2012; Vaugh, 2014; Wolff et al., 2015). This effect has been documented in varied psychological outcomes as well as related outcomes like emotional and sexual abuse of children (Millett, 2016).

While it is essential for mental health providers working with Latinx clients to recognize the extensive evidence of resilience among US Latinx people generally and Latinx immigrants specifically, there is a danger in relying too heavily on research studies that support these paradoxes. Some research, in fact, that has focused on the mental health of immigrant populations actually suggests *disadvantage*. For instance, in some studies, immigrants in general report a higher prevalence of conduct problems, phobias, and early substance use (Breslau et al., 2011) and decreased mental health functioning than their native-born ethnic counterparts (Farley, 2005). They may also display psychiatric disorder rates comparable to non-Latinx White subjects (Alegría et al., 2008). Overall, findings are inconsistent, and a review of the Immigrant Paradox and Hispanic Health Paradox literature bases suggests that health advantages do not apply evenly across ethnic groups, age groups, or genders, with, for example, Mexican American mothers at increased risk of adverse perinatal outcomes compared with other immigrant mothers (Gould et al., 2003; Teruya & Bazargan-Hejazi, 2013). Teruya and Bazargan-Hejazi, in conducting a review of extant literature, observe that immigrants who do not have health insurance, are older at time of migration, and those that have spent more time in the United States experience the worst outcomes (Teruya & Bazargan-Hejazi, 2013). Moreover, they state that "immigrant adolescents in general appear to be the most vulnerable to psychosocial stressors, with Latinx populations at greatest risk" (p. 501).

The latter may be accounted for, at least in part, by unprecedented increases in the migration of adolescents to the United States from Central America— particularly El Salvador, Guatemala, and Honduras—where crime, death, and violence have reached record levels. As previously noted, many of these adolescents may arrive as unaccompanied minors, seeking refuge in the United States following increases in crime victimization in Central America (Hiskey et al., 2016). The unprecedented danger in Central America was been cited as a "humanitarian emergency" by US President Barak Obama, with children and families being described as requiring "special attention" (Declaration by the Government of the United States of America and the Government of the United Mexican States Concerning Twenty-First Century Border Management, 2010) and "particular focus" (Federal Strategic Action Plan on Services for Victims of Human Trafficking in the United States, 2014) by several government agencies. Unsurprisingly, high rates of trauma exposure and posttraumatic stress are evident in recent waves of Central American youth migrants and their parents (Mercado et al., 2020; Venta & Mercado, 2019).

Research in other immigrant groups has also demonstrated that individuals who are displaced due to violence in society, abuse in the home, persecution, or deprivation are at a higher risk for developing psychopathology (Ehntholt & Yule, 2006; Fazel et al., 2012; Reed et al., 2012). These experiences distinguish many recent Hispanic immigrants from individuals who immigrated freely to the United States. Indeed, studies examining psychopathology in Hispanic adolescent immigrants in the United States confirm high rates of psychopathology (Locke et al., 1996; Perreira & Ornelas, 2013; Potochnick & Perreira, 2010) and suggest that the Immigrant Paradox and Hispanic Paradox may not apply. Likewise, a review of risk and protective factors for mental health in youth who are displaced from their home countries and resettled in high-income countries after immigration links high rates of adversity during migration and in their home country with related increases in posttraumatic stress, internalizing problems, and social maladjustment (Fazel et al., 2012). Across the literature on this topic, exposure to pre-migration violence, being female, migrating without a guardian, perceived discrimination after migration, exposure to post-migration violence, changes of residence after migration, parental exposure to violence, limited financial means, single-parent families, and parental psychopathology were identified as risk factors for immigrant youth mental health (Fazel et al., 2012). High parental/familial support, self-reported peer support, positive school experiences, and placement with a foster care family of the same ethnic background emerged as protective factors in this review (Fazel et al., 2012). In sum, across literatures related to Latinx and non-Latinx immigrants as well as youth and adult immigrants, the relation between immigration and mental health is inconsistent. Relations identified in prior research appear to depend on exposure to contextual risk factors as well as individual variables and preexisting vulnerability (e.g., exposure to violence in home country) rather than suggesting uniform health advantage for Hispanics or Immigrants. Indeed, structural factors exist that affect mental health in the immigrant community, such as immigration policies that increase stress and decrease access to healthcare. Social determinants of health inequality, income inequities, discrimination, and racial disparities in health outcomes continue to affect the health of immigrants (Castaneda et al., 2015).

THE NEED FOR CULTURALLY SENSITIVE PRACTICE

The clinical work with Latinx persons and immigrant populations has become a growing practice given the increase in the Latinx and immigrant populations in the United States. Therefore, it is important to understand cultural dynamics and important characteristics of Latinx cultures in the clinical setting. The United States is currently home to approximately 46.2 million immigrants (US Census Bureau, 2021), and a current estimate of the undocumented population is 11.4 million (US Department of Homeland Security, 2021). Certainly, even among non-immigrants, cultural variation exists. Culturally diverse individuals face an array of obstacles when seeking mental health treatment. A literature review of the past 15 years noted that individuals from ethnic minority groups face a number of barriers to mental healthcare such as accessibility, availability, and appropriateness (Turner et al., 2016), which may include communication issues, lack of trust, therapist bias, and no or limited insurance coverage of treatment. At the most basic level, if a clinician does not speak Spanish and is working with a monolingual Spanish-speaker, the language barrier could hamper the relationship with the client and contribute to client drop-out (Turner et al., 2016). Chapter 6 of this book will review working with interpreters and how to navigate this important area.

A significant and mounting concern in research and clinical practice has been the underutilization of mental health services among Latinx people. The US Latinx population has grown rapidly, and evidence suggests they are not receiving needed mental health services (Kouyoumdjian, Zamboanga, & Hansen, 2003). The absence of adequate services is even more troubling given recent events including the COVID-19 pandemic, racism, and policy changes that may disproportionately affect the mental health of Latinx and other culturally diverse communities. Kouyoumdjian and colleagues (2003) highlight that the within-group variability of Latinx persons, such as socioeconomic status, acculturation, and acculturative stress, may be associated with unique life experiences that influence mental health utilization rates in this population. Additionally, the authors further shed light into barriers to mental health utilization based on socioeconomic, cultural, and psychotherapeutic factors that contribute to the underutilization of mental health services with Latinx groups. For example, poor socioeconomic status has been linked to number of challenges to access to care despite elevated rates of depression within this population (Kouyoumdjian et al., 2003). In addition, perceptions of mental illness, including stigma, and some Latinx cultural values like *fatalimso*, *spirituality*, and *familismo* have been associated with underutilization of mental healthcare. Last, psychotherapeutic factors that continue to contribute to underutilization of mental health treatment include client–therapist mismatching, over reliance on Westernized interventions, and lack of culturally responsive assessment methods (Kouyoumdjian et al., 2003).

Beyond these barriers, there is a well-documented lack of culturally and linguistically sensitive mental health treatments for Latinx persons (Turner et al., 2016). To abate this problem in mental health treatment, it is essential to provide culturally sensitive, evidenced-based interventions to ethnically diverse clients. It is critical that clinicians and trainees begin to utilize cultural psychotherapy frameworks (La Roche, 2013) to effectively deliver evidenced-based interventions and provide effective and holistic psychological assessments. Previous research conducted by Miranda et al. (2005) has highlighted that culturally adapted interventions are effective; however, efficacy studies have not identified to what extent an intervention needs to be adapted to guide the treatment of individuals from ethnic minority groups. Many specialized treatment modalities have not undergone cultural adaptation for Latinx persons, and therefore Latinx people do not have access to the same breadth of services available to those who are non-Latinx. Mercado and Hinojosa (2017) attempted to fill this gap in specialized treatment modalities with Latinx and immigrant groups. For example, dialectical behavior therapy (DBT) has proved effective across clinical groups as an empirically supported treatment, but it has limited research in ethnic minority groups and was developed with majority non-Latinx participants. Mercado and Hinojosa (2017) offered a culturally adapted DBT modality to Latinx clients in South Texas and noted that, when delivered in a culturally responsive manner, a reduction in mental health symptoms and improved interpersonal functioning occurs. The authors incorporated Latinx cultural values in DBT's skills and interventions with a Latina adult client diagnosed with anxiety and depression. This study was one attempt to increase cultural competency and offered new knowledge to other healthcare providers regarding how to deliver DBT in a culturally sensitive manner, thus contributing to the reduction of healthcare disparities in Latinx groups.

In addition to interventions, there is a critical need for appropriate psychological assessment and evaluation with culturally diverse populations. Many clients in clinical settings have been misdiagnosed and labeled as a result of psychological evaluations that failed to conceptualize their symptoms and behaviors via a cultural lens. For instance, providers may inadvertently select and administer measures that are not meant to be administered to certain cultural groups or utilize measure that lack evidence supporting validity and reliability with the cultural group in question. This type of assessment practice can lead to misdiagnosis and clinical recommendations that are not culturally situated. In the most serious cases, this practice can lead to recommendations that may include psychopharmacological interventions that are not needed or even harmful. As clinical psychologists working with Latinx populations and members of other cultural groups, it is important to further our knowledge of psychological assessment to include appropriate psychological measures that will aid in diagnostic formulation and individualized clinical recommendations. This book attempts to be a resource of clinical utility for psychologists and other mental health practitioners working with the Latinx community by outlining best practices when working with this cultural group.

ETHICAL PRINCIPLES OF MENTAL HEALTH PRACTITIONERS

Exploring ethical standards of mental health professionals when working with Latinx groups is critical because they provide guiding principles when working with culturally diverse groups. For example, the American Psychological Association's (APA) Ethical Principles of Psychologists and Codes of Conduct highlight the importance of culture, individual, and role differences when working with clients (APA's Ethics Code, 2017). For instance, Standard 9, Assessment, mentions using psychological instruments for which validity and reliability have been established with members of the population being tested; we will discuss more about this standard in Chapter 5. Nonetheless, it also highlights that when validity and reliability are not available, discussing the strengths and limitations of the results and interpretation is imperative. Additionally, this standard indicates that using assessments that are appropriate to an individual's language preference is critical. In 1988, the APA's Board of Ethnic Minority Affairs attempted to provide guidelines for providers of psychological services to ethnic, linguistic, and culturally diverse populations. The task force devoted to this endeavor provided nine guidelines intended to be aspirational. The first indicated that psychologists should provide education about what psychological interventions entail; second, that psychologists should be aware of extant research in the population being served; and, third, that psychologists should recognize ethnicity and culture as core factors in the psychological assessment process. The next three standards encompass family, religion, and client language preference. The seventh guiding principle encourages incorporating the impact of adverse social, political, and environmental factors when working with culturally diverse populations. The eighth covers clinician biases and prejudice, and the last principle illustrates the importance of documenting culturally appropriate information in the records.

Much of the research addressing multicultural guidelines in the delivery of psychological services focuses on counseling interventions, where authors throughout the years have explored and shared culturally responsive and competent counseling interventions. An evident lack of research and clinical guidelines for psychological assessment across culturally diverse populations exists. A most recent attempt to address the scarcity of practical and clear guidelines for psychological testing was a joint monograph project developed by the Council of National Psychological Associations for the Advancement of Ethnic Minority Interests in 2016. This group included collaborations by ethnic minority psychological associations that included the Latinx, Asian, Black, and Indian psychological associations in addition to the APA, and the APA's Division 45, the Society for the Psychological Study of Culture, Ethnicity, and Race. This monograph, "Testing and Assessment with Persons & Communities of Color," is an important document that highlights testing and psychological considerations for African American, American Indian, Asian American, and Latinx persons. It provides brief but critical recommendations on managing issues of cultural diversity in the practice of psychology.

The APA updated and published its Multicultural Guidelines in 2017, where Guideline 9—"Psychologists strive to conduct culturally appropriate and informed research, teaching, supervision, consultation, assessment, interpretation, diagnosis, dissemination, and evaluation of efficacy as they address the first four levels of the *Layered Ecological Model of the Multicultural Guidelines*"—highlights the critical role psychologists play in acknowledging that assessment tools have the potential to mischaracterize and misrepresent the behavioral health needs of culturally diverse groups (Clauss-Ehlers et al., 2019). Moreover, APA's recently published *Guidelines on Race and Ethnicity in Psychology*, approved in August

2019, also include a guideline stressing the role of race, culture, and language in psychological assessment and clinical interventions. Guideline 9 states that "Psychologist strive to provide assessment, intervention, and consultation free from the negative effects of racial and ethnocultural bias." The APA task force also stressed how psychometric properties of assessments are a collection of scores of samples; thus, the reliability and validity of psychological instruments are often not established for racial and ethnic minority populations, and these groups are not well-represented even when they are included in some measures. They add that demonstrating cultural responsiveness in assessment includes addressing these limitations and documenting potential bias and its meaning for interpretive validity. Both APA guidelines address the importance of our intended goal for this book.

Similarly, the Council of Social Work Education highlights related culture and diversity core competencies (e.g., Engaging Diversity and Difference in Practice [Competency 2]; Advancing Human Rights and Social, Economic, and Environmental Justice [Competency 3]; and Assessing Individuals, Families, Groups, and Organizations, and Communities [Competency 7]; see Council of Social Work Education, 2022). Additionally, the National Association of Social Workers' ethical principles illustrate a commitment to social justice, such as supporting change initiatives that empower oppressed people, as well as cultural competence and demonstrating the skills in the provision of culturally informed services, including cultural humility (National Association of Social Workers, 2021). It is recommended that other mental health professionals, such as counselors, social workers, and psychiatrists, refer to their pertinent ethical codes of conduct that also support and guide multicultural and anti-oppressive practice.

PSYCHOLOGICAL ADVOCACY

The APA has played a pivotal role in advocacy, both in the practice of psychology and advancing science and in the dissemination of science related to working with culturally and disadvantaged groups. One recent example was the creation of a Chief Advocacy Officer and a committee devoted to furthering APA's broader advocacy efforts in nongovernmental sectors as well as amplifying the voice of psychology in Congress. The APA has also been instrumental in furthering knowledge that affects those who are disenfranchised through, for example, social advocacy movements on the effects of deep poverty led by Dr. Rosie Phillips (APA Deep Poverty Initiative, 2019) and immigration initiatives lead by Dr. Melba Vasquez (APA Presidential Task Force on Immigration, 2013). When addressing issues of advocacy at the national level, it is recommended that efforts be centralized and unified as there are times when many advocacy initiatives are spread throughout the various divisions, offices, and committees of APA and efforts are duplicated. In those instances, it is an arduous task to see what each entity at APA is doing. The National Latinx Psychological Association (NLPA) is another organization for Latinx mental health advocacy. Currently, a Special

Interest Group at NLPA, the Undocumented Collaborative has been formed to work on such endeavors. Specifically, a task force has been working on enhancing knowledge on best practices with immigration evaluations and working effectively with immigrant groups including Deferred Action for Childhood Arrivals (DACA) recipients as the fate of the program has come into question numerous times. This task force is just one of many efforts at NLPA designed to increase advocacy and knowledge regarding critical issues affecting those who are disadvantaged, particularly within the Latinx community. The Latinx Immigrant Health Alliance (LIHA) is a more recent multidisciplinary group that emerged from NLPA to support immigrant health research and advocacy. LIHA played a significant role in highlighting the psychological effects of anti-immigration policies in the United States, and Dr. Mercado presented his research findings and clinical work on the needs of Latinx children amid a global pandemic to the US Congressional Hispanic Caucus. Both authors of this book, Dr. Mercado and Dr. Venta, are co-founders of LIHA. State psychological associations are other entities where advocacy can also be enacted and perhaps serve more of an immediate need in emergent circumstances. For example, McAllen, Texas, was ground zero for family separations and is where the Texas Psychological Association (TPA) quickly took steps to assist in disseminating a science-based statement on the short- and long-term effects of family separation. The American Academy of Pediatrics, Human Rights Committee of Association of Social Workers, and many other associations also made public statements. Members were mobilized for media engagement and provided support on the Texas–Mexico border. Additionally, divisions and special interest groups of larger associations, such as the Social Justice Division and Diversity Division at TPA collaboratively worked on initiatives supporting similar endeavors. These include the United We Dream in Washington, DC, to generate a mental health initiative and resource list for states with DACA recipients who were under stress when the DACA program was rescinded by the Trump administration in 2017 and subsequently reviewed by the US Supreme Court (which ultimately did not rescind DACA). Other professional associations, like the Association of Behavioral and Cognitive Therapies, has a Latinx Special Interest Group that supports research and clinical work with Hispanic populations and the Society for Social Work and Research (SSWR) with Latinx Communities. Psychological advocacy like what we have just described is one way that psychologists, other mental health practitioners, and their associations can address the mental health needs of Latinx communities.

CULTURALLY INFORMED
PSYCHOLOGICAL ASSESSMENT

Undoubtedly, Latinx and many other minority groups are rising populations in the United States, with Latinx people being the largest minority group. These advances in diversity require test developers and users to attend to demographic characteristics of both the people for whom a test was developed and the increasing diversity of clinicians who use them. Performance and test scores can differ significantly between culturally diverse groups and the normed population, given the lack of diversity in standardization. For instance, a vocabulary test in English will more likely be an arduous task for someone whose primary language is not English. In this case, it is important not to compare this person with English-speaking norms as it will be a misrepresentation of their ability. There has been a rise in multicultural attention in psychological assessment, but the quality and quantity of research does not match the current need for information. Studies on culturally diverse groups are scarce for many popular psychological measures, ranging from the well-researched Personality Assessment Inventory (PAI), to projective techniques like the Thematic Apperception Test (Miller & Loveler, 2020). Chapter 5 will explore psychological measurements that are commonly used with the Latinx population.

The need for multicultural research in psychological assessment is critical and needed now more than ever due to our existing and growing diverse society and in specific regions in our country. For example, practicing in a border community, we have seen a rise in unaccompanied minors and immigrant mothers and their children crossing the Rio Grande, which forms the border between Northern Mexico and Texas. This is a distinct region in the United States, one that is a predominantly occupied by the Latinx community and represents the meeting of many immigrant groups and cultures (Mercado et al., 2022). Due to these diverse demographics, psychologists and mental health professionals are increasingly serving immigrant children and adults, documented and undocumented, who are presenting with a multitude of problems across settings including schools, clinics, hospitals, and prisons (Casas, 2017). Thus, clinicians should be aware of this important population as practitioners and researchers in an increasingly multicultural society.

The Latinx community has experienced ongoing sociopolitical stressors for decades, and this has intensified over the past couple of years due to the recent political climate in the United States. For example, incidents of racism, discrimination, colorism, and anti-immigrant sentiment at different levels of US society have negatively affected the psychological and social well-being of Latinx persons (Casas & Cabrera, 2011). Thus, it is imperative that psychological assessment practices also address sociocultural factors when working with Latinx clients. Inadequate and biased psychological assessment can result in misdiagnosis, inappropriate treatment, and further healthcare disparities among this population and may perpetuate what it intends to mitigate. Therefore, it is critical that psychologists be aware of the limitations of psychological batteries, the assessment process, and their own biases when working with Latinx groups.

In previous psychological models highlighting sources of error in the diagnosis process, like the Brunswick Lens Model (Wing, 1980), culture was not specifically highlighted as a factor affecting the reliability and validity of the assessment and diagnostic process. We now know that not including culture as a core factor in the assessment process increases the likelihood of misdiagnosis or pathologizing of normal behavior, such as historical events, like the *Larry P. v. Riles* (1979) case, which highlighted the issue of discrimination in psychological testing and bias when assessing Black children in the education system who were misdiagnosed with intellectual disabilities. This practice led to the misplacement of black children in special education programs, stigma, inadequate education, and failure to nurture in those children the skills necessary to thrive. The courts agreed that the defendants used standardized intelligence tests that were racially and culturally biased and, in turn, had a discriminatory impact on Black children. One of the most difficult problems in psychological testing is that some ethnic groups obtain lower average scores on some psychological tests; most controversially, African Americans score about 15 points lower than White Americans on standardized intelligence tests (Kaplan & Saccuzzo, 2013). Some psychologists believe that test developers must try to find selection procedures that will end all discriminatory practices and protect the interests of minority group members (Kaplan & Saccuzzo, 2013). To reduce and eliminate similar issues in psychological testing, Kaplan and Saccuzzo (2013) proposed two avenues to ameliorate test bias, including eliminating psychological testing or developing tailored psychological measures for each cultural group. Given the arduous task at hand and the need for psychological testing in the assessment process, it is pivotal to understand the role of culture in the case conceptualization of clients and the decision-making process of selecting adequate psychological instruments when working with culturally diverse populations, including Latinx groups. This book is one attempt to capture and address the practical challenges in trying to provide culturally responsive psychological assessment to Latinx groups.

CONCLUSION

We began with an introduction of the diversity of the Latinx and immigrant populations in the United States and the need for culturally informed psychological assessments. The ethical implications of psychological testing and assessment and the role of psychological advocacy were discussed. The remainder of this book is organized into seven chapters. The first three chapters highlight Latinx cultural values in the context of psychological assessment. Chapter 1 clarifies the difference between cultural competency and cultural humility in the testing context, while Chapter 2 examines the role of Latinx cultural values in relation to assessment. Chapter 3 discusses clinical interviewing and the critical need for cultural conceptualization when working with clients in mental health settings. Chapter 4 explores psychometric issues in assessment with Latinx people, and there we review the Culture Language Interpretive Matrix, cross-cultural psychometrics, and cultural bias in commonly used tools. The chapter also discusses the importance of understanding the psychometrics of instruments used with culturally diverse groups. Chapter 5 covers psychological instruments commonly used with the Latinx population in clinical settings. Cognitive and personality measures are included, in addition to specialized instruments for assessing trauma symptoms and assessing Latinx youth. Chapter 6 covers troubleshooting scenarios that some psychologists and other mental health practitioners may encounter, ranging from working with interpreters, barriers to treatment that Latinx persons encounter, and how to deal with microaggressions in the assessment process. The chapter also includes clinical considerations when working with immigrant groups, and we conclude in Chapter 7 by offering future directions in psychological assessment with culturally diverse populations.

1

Cultural Humility in the Testing Context

Cultural humility in the therapeutic alliance in psychotherapy has been studied extensively but in the psychological assessment and testing context much is yet to be explored. Many definitions of cultural humility have been put forth. Hook et al. (2013) noted that cultural humility involves intrapersonal (such as a self-examination of cultural bias) and interpersonal components while being open to others' cultural background and nurturing mutual respect. Hook et al. (2013) found that cultural humility was viewed as desirable by clients, was related to significant improvement in symptoms, and contributed to solid therapeutic alliance. Foronda et al. (2016) defined cultural humility as a "process of openness, self-awareness, being egoless, and incorporating self-reflection and critique after willingly interacting with diverse individuals" (Foronda et al., 2016, p. 210). Possible outcomes the authors note include mutual empowerment, respect, and lifelong learning. Additionally, Mosher, Hook, Captari, Davis, DeBlaere, and Owen (2017), provided a cultural humility therapeutic framework for engaging culturally diverse clients in psychotherapy. They stressed the importance of engaging in critical self-examination and self-awareness, focusing on the therapeutic alliance, repairing cultural ruptures, and navigating value differences in psychotherapy in service of cultural humility.

Cultural humility is not a new concept in the psychological testing context, although it has not thoroughly been explored and investigated either. Dr. Israel Cuellar, a pioneer in the cultural diversity movement in psychological assessment, highlighted cultural variables such as cultural orientation, cultural identity, and acculturation in the psychological assessment of Latinx persons (Cuellar, 1998). Dr. Cuellar emphasized that ignoring such variables can decrease the reliability and validity of testing, with negative implications for the meaningful interpretation of psychological test findings. Just as culture has an impact on the manifestations of psychological symptoms, culture also has an impact on psychological data. It is imperative to look beyond the data as presented in a norm-based context and instead interpret data via a cultural lens. The psychological community, as reflected in revisions made in the *Diagnostic and Statistical Manual of Mental Disorders*

(DSM-5), has emphasized the importance of culture in diagnostic formulations. For example, the additions of the Cultural Formulation Interview (CFI) and the World Health Organization Disability Assessment Schedule 2.0 (WHODAS 2.0) to the DSM-5, enhance its clinical utility and allow a more global assessment of functioning. Both of these resources may be used to avoid misdiagnosis of Latinx and other culturally diverse populations.

The National Institutes of Health defines cultural humility as "a lifelong process of self-reflection and self-critique, whereby the individual not only learns about another's culture, but starts with the examination with his or her own beliefs and cultural identities" (Hogg Foundation for Mental Health, 2021). This process allows us to learn about other cultures yet highlights the need for self-reflection on our values, beliefs, and multiple identities and how these personal factors can impact the assessment process. For example, having assessed clients from Central and South America, Asian countries, and European countries, we have realized the essential role of understanding and reflecting on our own cultural beliefs and cultural identities as clinicians before we can understand the role of culture in the psychological symptoms of others. This learning process is essential if we are to minimize clinician bias in the assessment of people of color, including Latinx groups. A clinician without awareness of their own cultural identities and values may inadvertently minimize certain client symptoms and overpathologize other salient symptoms that are culturally sanctioned. The mental status exam and clinical interview can be easily conducted through a biased lens, leading to a clinical diagnosis that is impressionistic, rather than based on strict adherence to diagnostic criteria. These errors will undoubtedly affect the working alliance and the assessment process with people of color and lead to misdiagnosis. In other words, culture must play a key role in case conceptualization for every client, including those undertaking psychological testing. Simply having some "cultural competence" is not enough. Cultural humility is closely related to cultural competence, but significant differences exist and are important to understand.

Cultural competence measures one's knowledge of other cultures, but it does not reflect our own cultural background, of which consideration is needed for an appropriate and ethical psychological assessment. In fact, the American Psychological Association (APA) recently published three different guidelines that highlight the importance of cultural self-awareness. For example, Guideline 2 in the Multicultural Guidelines (2017) indicates that "Psychologists aspire to recognize and understand that as cultural beings, they hold attitudes and beliefs, that can influence their perceptions of and interactions with others, as well as their clinical and empirical conceptualizations. As such, psychologists strive to move beyond conceptualizations rooted in categorical assumptions, biases and/ or formulations, based on limited knowledge about individual and communities." In the *APA Guidelines on Race and Ethnicity in Psychology* (2019), Guideline 3 notes that "Psychologists strive for awareness of their own positionality in relation to ethnicity and race," which requires awareness of oneself as cultured and cultural humility. These guidelines emphasize the role of self-awareness, which includes a deeper understanding of the way culture and race/ethnicity have shaped our own worldviews and values including norms, practices, and communication patterns. These experiences can include racial inequities or privilege. This type of self-recognition, continued self-evaluation, and commitment to act to "redress the power imbalance in relationships and systems" is known as *cultural humility* (APA, 2017). Another pertinent and relevant APA Guideline in *Race and Ethnicity in Psychology* (2019) that furthers our understanding of cultural humility in the testing context (including case conceptualization) is Guideline 10, where "psychologists strive to engage in reflective practice by exploring how their worldviews and positionalities may affect the quality and range of psychological services they provide." This guideline highlights how reflective practices increase awareness of the effects of our biases on our practice and how these biases may affect our clinical judgment during psychological assessment. For example, psychologists should think critically about what they are doing, why they are doing it, and how they are doing it (APA, 2019). Thus, cultural humility helps with checking the power imbalances that exist in the dynamics of a psychologist–client relationship.

Teaching cultural humility may be an arduous endeavor; nonetheless, research surrounding cultural humility and the training of future psychologists highlights creative ways of developing cultural competence and cultural humility (Tormala, Patel, Soukup, & Clarke, 2018). Tormala and colleagues (2018) utilized the cultural formulation outline of the DSM-5 in an innovative way to deepen cultural awareness and humility in trainees. The authors explored cultural humility in individual supervision with trainees, didactic instruction, and during formal class delivery. The Cultural Humility Scale (CHS) is a method of measuring cultural humility in the therapeutic alliance (Hook et al., 2013). The CHS includes 12 items that highlight respect, openness, and being genuine, which the client completes. Measuring one's cultural humility is important to examine how we see culture in self-examination and self-awareness. This can be further explored and examined in supervision. Because cultural humility is difficult to teach using traditional methods like classroom lectures, another creative way of developing cultural humility in trainees and healthcare professionals is to prompt reflective journaling (Schuessler et al., 2012). Using a qualitative design, Schuessler and colleagues (2012) explored more than 200 journal entries that included critical thinking and self-reflection on practice. Their results indicated that reflections, over time, contributed to the development of cultural humility (Schuessler et al., 2012). Additionally, Hook et al. (2013) proposed that the clinical supervisor plays a key role in the development of cultural humility by building a strong relationship with culturally diverse supervisees and also by modeling cultural humility him- or herself. The supervisor can engage trainees from a culturally humble perspective by adopting an initiative-invite-still-approach (Hook et al., 2013) which helps make culture a welcome supervisory focus in conversations and invites trainees to freely and fully engage. Another way clinical supervisors can aid in developing cultural humility in their students is through cultivating relevant outside activities and experiences. For example, facilitating a service-learning component to course delivery in undergraduate and graduate courses (including reflective journaling on their experiences) can further cultural awareness and humility. Another activity that highlights cultural humility is the use of cultural autobiography, a method that the authors have applied. It has been a very well accepted activity among students who get an opportunity to focus on the influence culture has played in the development of their identity, self-concept, and other life goals. Since culture is a broad construct, students incorporate ethnicity, race, gender, sexual orientation, religion and/or spirituality, family contexts, nationality, and any other factors they choose into their autobiographies, deciding which aspect(s) of culture they would like to include.

Participating in hands-on research that includes foci on cultural diversity and social justice can also enhance cultural humility for trainees while dovetailing with their other training goals (e.g., research, publication, face-to-face hours). For instance, trainees working with Dr. Mercado have volunteered their time at a local Humanitarian Respite Center near the Texas–Mexico border. The respite center is a place where recently immigrated families and refugees arrive (after processing by immigration officials) before their departure to their sponsors anywhere across the United States. Families are there temporarily—for a few hours to a day or two. Students have an opportunity to volunteer with the daily operations of the center, including cleaning, food preparation and serving, distributing hygiene and clothing items, assisting center workers, and sometimes playing with the children. The students also have an opportunity to interact with the families and talk to them, particularly within the confines of the aforementioned service work and if data collection is ongoing. The families are from all over Central and South America and some are from Africa, Asia, and beyond. It is during those interactions and experiences, in addition to reflective journaling assignments, that students are able to reflect on their experiences and evaluate their cultural humility in a unique way. These experiences are broadly based on the contact hypothesis that encourages students to connect with people who are different from them and encourages them to have positive experiences (Hook et al., 2013). These unique experiences are always met with gratitude from students who are thankful for an opportunity to compassionately and respectfully respond to the needs expressed by the families they serve, an experience students say they will always remember and will likely impact their provision of psychological services in the future.

In the clinical supervision realm with graduate students and trainees, in addition to the self-assessment and related activities described above, trainees should also be observed for cultural humility via verbal cues and behaviors, including nonverbal signals in the assessment setting. Having advanced technology and recording equipment facilitates this learning opportunity, as does in vivo supervision during an assessment session. Through video, trainees also have the opportunity to observe themselves during session to explore those behaviors that indicate cultural humility and those that did not. For instance, behaviors that indicate cultural humility in the assessment process with a client can include asking details about the client's story and what is important to them as well as displaying genuine interest in knowing that information. Other techniques demonstrating cultural humility include asking open-ended questions; focusing on cultural background to include values, customs, traditions, and communicate respect; and being honest regarding a lack of understanding or desire to understand the client's background. Another effective reading assignment given to psychology trainees and psychiatry residents during my career as a psychologist has been the book *Crazy Like Us: The Globalization of the American Psyche*, by Ethan Watters (2010). It details specific encounters across the globe and discusses the role of mental health and culture and the manifestations of mental health in different cultural groups. Behaviors that may not support the development of cultural humility in the psychological evaluation process include relying on a structured clinical interview, utilizing a set agenda that does not allow for flexibility, not focusing on what the client wants to divulge, cutting off the client, not listening, ignoring the client's culture and other aspects of their identity, making assumptions about the client's cultural background, and making statements that do not respect the client's background. The supervision experience is one way to explore cultural humility and discuss the supervisee's progress (or lack thereof) in demonstrating cultural humility in session. Doing so should be integrated into the trainee's supervision plan, with targeted and measurable goals to gauge and monitor behaviors, from both the trainee's and supervisor's perspectives, during the assessment session to address the trainee's strengths and weaknesses. Including cultural humility in the supervision experience of trainees scaffolds proper development of both cultural competency and humility.

Overall, cultural competency and cultural humility are distinct and essential avenues to expand our effectiveness in the psychological assessment process. One aspect of developing competency and cultural humility in assessment is understanding culturally diverse groups' values, norms, and unique characteristics that play a role in the assessment process, such as in case conceptualization and deciding which appropriate psychological instruments are best suitable for the assessment at hand (this will be further discussed in Chapter 5). Also, as psychologists and/or other mental health practitioners, it is critical to develop a multicultural orientation in supervision and assure that culture is also a central focus in the clinical supervision experience with trainees. Integrating a multicultural framework in clinical supervision is one way to help trainees develop cultural humility (Hook et al., 2013). Incorporating a multicultural framework in supervision can be done no matter what clinical supervision model is being employed. Adding multicultural and cultural humility elements such as trainee's integration of the CFI (discussed in Chapter 3), cultural humility assignments, and other related supervision activities to the student evaluation and trainee plan can formalize this critical experience.

2
—

Understanding Latinx Cultural Perspectives in Relation to Assessment

This chapter highlights the importance of incorporating Latinx cultural values in the psychological assessment process.

LATINX CULTURAL VALUES

Although Latinx persons in the United States fall under the umbrella terms "Latinx/Latinos" or "Hispanics," as discussed previously, even a cursory look will reveal within and between group differences in this heterogeneous group of Caribbean, South American, Central American, European, and Mexican individuals, as we discussed in the Introduction. Importantly, heterogeneity within Latinx people, particularly regarding their adherence to Latinx cultural values, explains to some extent differing perceptions of mental health. Cultural beliefs such as *fatalismo*, which holds that life is not under one's immediate control, and *familismo*, which highlights family unity, can, respectively, prompt a sense of resignation as opposed to solution seeking and result in denigrating one's health needs to promote family well-being (Caldwell, Couture, & Nowotny, 2008). Alternatively, *familismo* can form a pathway to social support (Abate, Bailey, & Venta, 2022). *Machismo* and *caballerismo*, the male obligation to care for and defend the family, and *marianismo*, the obligation of females to consider the needs of the family prior to their own needs, may result in similar self-effacing action and choices (Caldwell et al., 2008). The cultural values noted above may affect the acceptability of accessing mental healthcare for Latinx clients and may also influence the stigma associated with receiving such care (Satcher, 2001). The assessment of these cultural values and gender roles is critical in evaluation. A cultural clinical interview may collect ample information, however, specific measures may also aid in the evaluation process. The Traditional Machismo and Caballerismo

Scale (TMCS) is a 20-item instrument that measures these two aspects of gender role expectations among Mexican American men: traditional *machismo* (i.e., in a family, a father's wish is law) and *caballerismo* (i.e., men hold their mothers and females in high regard) (Arciniega et al., 2008). While the traditional *machismo* subscale focuses on hypermasculinity, aggression, emotional avoidance, and antisocial behavior, the *caballerismo* subscale focuses on emotional connectedness, respect, and duty to family. *Marianismo* encompasses the traditional values of Latina femininity and emphasizes culturally valued qualities such as interpersonal harmony, inner strength, self-sacrifice, and morality (Castillo et al. 2010). Castillo et al. (2010) developed and validated the Marianismo Belief Scale. This scale of 24 items consists of five subscales that assess the extent (strongly agree to strongly disagree) to which a Latina believes she should enculturate and practice the cultural values that comprise the construct of marianismo. First, the Family Pillar subscale is the belief that Latinas are the main source of strength for the family and are responsible for keeping the family unified and happy (i.e., "A Latina keeps the family unified"). Second, the Virtuous and Chaste subscale reflects the belief that Latinas should be morally pure in thought and sexuality (i.e., "A Latina should remain a virgin until marriage"). Third, the Subordinate to Other subscale emphasizes the belief that Latinas must show obedience and respect for the Latinx hierarchical power structure (i.e., "A Latina must satisfy her partner's sexual needs without argument"). Fourth, the Self-silencing to Maintain Harmony subscale reflects the belief that Latinas should not share personal thoughts or needs in order to maintain harmony in relationships (i.e., "A Latina should not express her needs to her partner"). Last, the Spiritual Pillar subscale reflects the belief that Latinas are the spiritual leaders of the family and are responsible for the family's spiritual growth (i.e., "A Latina is the spiritual leader of the family"). Castillo et al. (2010) noted good validity and evidence of the Marianismo Belief Scale being a multidimensional construct.

The cultural value of *familismo* is perhaps especially noteworthy in its effects on Latinx mental health help-seeking intentions. For instance, a hesitancy in obtaining treatment may be due to *familismo* and the shame that treatment-seeking may incur for the family or hesitancy in revealing private information regarding the family and concerns of ethnicity, immigration status, or racial stigmatization (Caldwell et al., 2008; Guarnaccia, Martinez, & Acosta, 2005). In a study by Villatoro, Morales, and Mays (2014), a particular facet of *familismo* represented by the level of perceived family support, or behavioral *familismo*, was studied for its effects on Latinx utilization of mental health services. Results indicated that high levels of perceived family support predicted use of alternative sources of mental healthcare (e.g., religious). In this case, the fact that the individual feels supported may reflect levels of enculturation in which not only *familismo* is strong but accompanying cultural values are as well (i.e., *curanderismo* and religiosity), likely resulting in benefits such as decreased stress and increased self-validation. The converse is also true, as a study by Miville and Constantine (2006) demonstrates: lower perceived familial social support contributes to positive help-seeking attitudes and behavior. The latter may reflect a negative family environment which creates an increased need for mental healthcare (Villatoro et al., 2014) or a perception of inadequate familial support. Social support generally, and perhaps more so family support for Latinx people, provides benefits which are widely recognized and noted.

A cultural clinical interview may collect ample data to determine the role that *familismo* has on the client being evaluated. However, if additional information and data are needed, *familismo* scales maybe used. For example, the Attitudinal Familism Scale (AFS) by Steidel and Contreras (2003) and the Familism Scale by Sabogal et al. (1987) are two widely used measures that may be employed to determine the level of *familismo* in the client being assessed.

Clinicians must recognize the importance of understanding the client's worldview, attitudes, and values in order to collaborate and adequately recommend what treatment approaches or assessments are necessary and will be deemed acceptable to the client. It is then critical to assess and integrate Latinx cultural values into practice to ultimately increase treatment engagement and retention (Edwards & Cardemil, 2015). In particular, understanding the variation of cultural values in Latinx clients and, specifically, the degree of *familismo*, *respeto* (respect), and *personalismo* in each Latinx client is important and can provide valuable information beyond language, ethnicity, and acculturation level (Rivera, 2008). However, relations between Latinx cultural values and mental health outcomes are not simple. In the case of *familismo*, for instance, evidence suggests that it can serve as a protective factor, buffering against significant mental health outcomes, but a greater sense of familial obligation may lead some Latinx persons to take on arduous family-oriented responsibilities, such as caretaking for elderly relatives or providing financial support to extended family members (Gloria, Ruiz, & Castillo, 2004). Some research has also suggested that high levels of *familismo* may contribute to family conflict and distress (Hernandez et al., 2010). *Personalismo*, on the other hand, refers to a practice that emphasizes politeness and courtesy and that helps establish good rapport and connection with a person. *Personalismo* is an unconditional recognition of the essential value of each individual and serves as the foundation of many other cultural values, like *confianza* (trust). In the Latinx culture, having *confianza*, having a trust based largely on personal relationships and rapport, the idea that a "person knows us," far outweighs the person's credentials and personal accomplishments. Therefore, without *confianza* a clinician is unlikely to have any significant success in working with the Latinx client in the assessment or intervention process. Therefore, mental health providers need to understand their clients' adherence and response to cultural values. It is critical for clinicians to probe beyond diagnostic clinical interviews—which usually include with demographics, history, background, presenting problem, and level of functioning across domains—to include a cultural clinical interview and/or appropriate measures of the client's adherence to cultural values.

Additionally, perceived appropriateness of psychological treatment and assessment can be impacted by religious or cultural views and thus alternative resources being sought out (i.e., a preacher or general practitioner, *curanderos*, or *sobadores*; Satcher, 2001; Office of the Surgeon General, National Institute of Mental Health,

2001). However, when such cultural practices are present, it is pivotal to respect and embrace it. The term *curandero* (male) or *curandera* (female) refers to the use of any form of folk-traditional healing, even though there may be significant differences between practices. Their skills include healing, herbalism, massage, prayer, card reading, midwifery, and spiritual cures (Clark, Bunik, & Johnson, 2010). Some *curanderos* practice only one skill, such as herbalism. Others practice a combination of skills. *Curanderos* practicing in the United States are commonly of Latinx ethnicity, in their mid-50s, married, and with no formal medical training. They have obtained special skills that have either been passed down by ancestral *curanderos* or taught through apprenticeships (Clark et al., 2010; Padilla et al., 2001; Tafur, Crowe, & Torres, 2009). Many *curanderos* practice out of their homes and receive donations in lieu of practice fees (Amerson, 2008; Padilla et al., 2001; Tafur et al., 2009). *Sobadores* specialize in massage. They tend to serve as popular chiropractors, who, without formal studies, heal pain by mixing body knowledge with traditional Mexican and herbal medicine. They use *sobada* (massage) to care for pulled muscles and injured joints, as well as to move internal organs. *Sobadores* are widely available and used as traditional healers by Mexican immigrants, Mexican Americans, and other Latinx communities in the United States. We have found that working alongside *curanderos*, such as shamans, especially in rural areas and underserved communities, contributes to a sense of trust and increases the utilization of psychological services.

It is critical to understand that there are cultural variations in emotional expression that may impact clinical work with the Latinx population. The *Diagnostic and Statistical Manual of Mental Disorders* (DSM-5) refers to *Cultural Concepts of Distress* (previously referred to as Culture-Bound Syndromes; American Psychiatric Association, 2013), or "ways that cultural groups experience, understand, and communicate suffering, behavioral problems, or troubling thoughts and emotions" (American Psychiatric Association, 2013, p. 758). The DSM-5 emphasizes three different types of cultural concepts are necessary to understand and document distress among diverse populations (American Psychiatric Association, 2013). These include cultural syndromes, cultural idioms of distress, and cultural explanations or perceived causes. One example of a relevant cultural concept of distress among immigrants of Latinx origin is "*Ataque de Nervios*" which is considered a "normative expressions of acute distress" that is characterized by "symptoms of intense emotional upset, including acute anxiety, anger, or grief; screaming and shouting uncontrollably; attacks of crying; trembling; heat in the chest rising to the head; [and] becoming verbally and physically aggressive [among other symptoms]" (American Psychiatric Association, 2013, p. 833). A generalized feature of *Ataque de Nervios* is a sense of being out of control, and the *Ataques* are often related to a stressful life event, mostly involving the family (e.g., family separation, death of a loved one). Some DSM disorders that have been linked to *Ataque de Nervios* include panic attacks, panic disorder, conversion disorder, unspecified or specified forms of dissociative disorders, and intermittent explosive disorder (American Psychiatric Association, 2013).

Another important cultural consideration for evaluators is to recognize so-matic symptoms that may differ from those traditionally reported by the general population (e.g., feeling pins and needles in your hands or feet, feeling heat inside the body, sensations of fluttering in the stomach) and which may reflect distress from a cultural perspective. Somatic disturbances are important symptoms to as-sess and document as they relate to Cultural Concepts of Distress, such as *Ataque de Nervios* and *Susto*.

In sum, the culturally relevant psychological evaluation process requires that evaluators integrate cultural factors into each step of the evaluation process, starting with assessment, continuing into the interpretation, and culminating in the diagnosis process. In the psychological assessment process, understanding Latinx cultural values and the cultural variations of emotional expression plays a critical role. It is therefore crucial that psychologists and other mental health practitioners include a cultural assessment to assess the degree and level of Latinx cultural values that are present in the client in order to adequately assess the client and individualize treatment recommendations.

ACCULTURATION IN PSYCHOLOGICAL ASSESSMENT

In the psychological assessment setting, it is important to examine the client's ac-culturation level to gauge the degree to which acculturation may or may not be an issue that may affect test results. A culturally competent clinician with a deep understanding of cultural humility will include acculturation in the case concep-tualization process to aid in developing appropriate clinical hypotheses and, ulti-mately, in deciding what psychological batteries are appropriate to use. In doing so, it is important to revisit and define acculturation.

As we discussed in the Introduction, a common explanation of acculturation refers to a bidimensional process in which an individual will range from high to low on affiliation with their host (post-migration) culture and, on a separate axis, from high to low on affiliation with their culture of origin (Sam & Berry, 2010). Individuals high in affiliation with their host culture and low in affiliation with their culture of origin, for instance, are described as "assimilated," whereas individuals high on both axes are referred to as "bicultural/integrated." Individuals low in both metrics are described as "marginalized," and individuals with high af-filiation with their culture of origin only are referred to as "traditional/separated." Overall, acculturation is conceptualized as a change in cultural identity, one that includes shifts in various cultural dimensions including typical practices, values, and identifications (Schwarz et al., 2010).

Literature regarding the link between acculturation and mental health is mixed, with some studies of the Immigrant Paradox reporting that lower acculturation with the host county accounts for health benefits (e.g., Kaplan & Marks, 1990) and others showing that low acculturation among immigrants is risk factor for nega-tive mental health outcomes (e.g., Hwang & Ting, 2008). Indeed, the aforemen-tioned Immigrant and Hispanic Paradox literatures cite that individuals with lower acculturation to the United States experience greater benefits (Teruya & Bazargan-Hejazi, 2013) and that some of the identified health benefits noted in the Paradox research erode with increasing time and generations in the United States as acculturation to US culture and damaging health behaviors (e.g., smoking) increases (Kondo, Rossi, Schwartz, Zamboanga, & Scalf, 2015). Numerous explanations have been put forth to explain these inconsistent findings, including heterogeneity within and across immigrant groups, inconsistent measurement of acculturation, and lack of measurement of related variables regarding ethnic identity (Bulut & Gayman, 2015). In studies that have endeavored to address these limitations, acculturation emerges as a complex construct without simple relations to mental health. Indeed, findings do not link simple conceptualizations of high or low acculturation to mental health but rather identify risk in specific interactions between both axes put forth by Sam and Berry (2010). Specifically, marginalization appears to be relatively consistently associated with negative mental health outcomes whereas integration is associated with positive mental health outcomes (Yoon et al., 2013). Support for this conclusion has been documented with regard to both Latinx and Asian immigrants (Bulut & Gayman, 2015).

Critiques of existing literature on acculturation in the context of mental health, however, have cited inconsistent measurement and definition of acculturation across studies (Bulut & Gayman, 2015; Teruya & Bazargan-Hejazi, 2013). Indeed, acculturation is often treated as though it is synonymous with acculturative stress—self-reported distress during the acculturation process (e.g., distress associated with speaking with an accent). Existing literature regarding acculturative stress is relatively consistent across Latinx groups, suggesting that distress while adjusting to acculturation has a negative impact on all ethnic groups' mental health (Caplan, 2007; Teruya & Bazargan-Hejazi, 2013; Turner, Lloyd, & Taylor, 2006) with particularly profound impacts on the substance use of Latins people in the United States (Turner et al., 2006). Relatedly, perceived racism and discrimination have been linked to negative mental health and academic outcomes in immigrant youth in the United States (Suárez-Orozco, Rhodes, & Milburn, 2009; Smokowski & Bacallao, 2006). In studies that account for both acculturation level and acculturative stress, the latter emerges as the significant risk factor for psychopathology (Hwang & Ting, 2008), indicating that experiences of perceived discrimination, including colorism (Breland-Noble, 2013) and related distress are more relevant to mental health in immigrant groups than cultural identification alone.

Acculturation Measures

The assessment of mental health disorders is often a complex and arduous process. This process is even more challenging when we include assessment of the client's cultural background, their life experiences, and the impact of acculturation on mental health symptoms and behaviors (Schraufnagel et al., 2006). Only a few multiethnic acculturation measures exist, such as the Vancouver Index of Acculturation (VIA; Ryder, Alden, & Paulhus, 2000), and most are culture-specific. One common measure used with Latinx persons is the Acculturation Rating Scale for Mexican Americans (ARSMA-II), a measure that was developed by Israel Cuellar in 1980 and revised in 1995. It is the most widely used acculturation measure, having been cited approximately 2,684 times since its development. It was designed as a bidimensional measure and contains two orientation subscales, Mexican Orientation Scale (MOS) and Anglo Orientation Scale (AOS; Cuellar, Arnold, & Maldonado, 1995). In the ARSMA-II, acculturation is measured by language spoken; the respondent's identification of culture in himself or herself, in his or her family, and in his or her friends; and the language involved in everyday activities. The ARSMA-II has been used extensively in research and can be used clinically. An alternative acculturation measure used with Latinx populations includes the Short Acculturation Scale for Hispanics (Marin et al., 1987), which consists of 12 items with validation criteria for respondent's generation, length of residence in the United States, age at arrival, ethnic-self-identification, and acculturation index. It has been shown to be a valid instrument for assessing acculturation among Latinx people (Ellison, Jandorf, & Duhamel, 2011). The ARSMA-II can provide acculturation data to guide the selection of specific therapeutic approaches.

3

Clinical Interviewing and Cultural Conceptualization

Another important resource that can be used to assess acculturation and cultural values (outside of acculturation measures like the Acculturation Rating Scale for Mexican-Americans [ARSMA-II; Cuellar et al., 1995]) is a thorough clinical interview that incorporates and highlights the client's culture. A *cultural clinical interview* is one of the most, if not *the* most, critical components of the psychological assessment process when working with a culturally diverse population like Latinx people. In many cases, a clinical interview is all that will be done, and, therefore, a thorough clinical interview and case conceptualization where culture is a central and core element is important. In clinical practice, making the distinction between psychopathological symptoms and culture-related experiences may be an arduous task for some clinicians. Paniagua (2005) identifies time limitations and managed care companies being barriers for effective assessment and treatment. Limited time with the culturally diverse client is a barrier in most cases, as Latinx persons may not open up in a first session—stigma and shame regarding mental health symptoms may prohibit them from reporting their emotional problems early in a therapeutic relationship. Additionally, current standard and most used clinical inventories and ratings scales do not focus on cultural variables, which may lead to an assessment that lacks specific cultural contexts (Paniagua, 2005). Therefore, in some circumstances, it is best to rely on a thorough culture clinical interview.

By having familiarity with ethnic identity models and using specific diagnostic interviewing and case formulation strategies, psychologists can approach conceptualization, diagnosis, and treatment planning in a more reflective and deliberate manner. For example, the Cultural Formulation Interview (CFI; APA, 2013) is one avenue of eliciting important information that aids in a culturally grounded case formulation. Although the *Diagnostic and Statistical Manual of Mental Disorders* (DSM-5) did face criticism due to repackaging of various disorders and the development of new ones without transparency and validity (Whooley, 2016), one positive addition to the DSM-5 is the emerging measures section and the clinical utility of the tools described in that section. One such assessment tool is the CFI, a cross-cultural assessment tool that was revised due to the shortcomings of the DSM-IV-TR's Outline for Cultural Formulation (OCF). The CFI field trial took place across 6 countries, 14 sites, and with 321 clients to examine its feasibility, acceptability, and clinical utility with both clients and clinicians (Aggarwal et al., 2013). The CFI highlights the inclusion of cultural factors in diagnostic formulations and treatment planning. Although some research on the CFI has mixed reviews (Aggarwal et al., 2013; Paralikar, Deskmukh, & Weiss, 2019; Ramirez-Stege &Yarris, 2017) other studies have documented its effectiveness in cultural competency among trainees (Mills et al., 2017). Despite the availability of cultural assessment tools like the CFI, many clinicians do not utilize the CFI or any cultural conceptualization models and therefore fail to include relevant cultural considerations when diagnosing and assessing clients. Clinical interviewing is a core element of the psychological assessment process. Thus, it is important to understand the different types of clinical interviews, such as structured, unstructured, or semi-structured, and their receptibility with Latinx clients.

CHOOSING THE ASSESSMENT METHOD

The Case of Antonio

Antonio is an 11-year-old boy from El Salvador. He and his mother emigrated to the United States to flee growing violence in their home country. His father was murdered by gangs after refusing multiple recruitment attempts. Antonio and his mother were also threatened with death if Antonio did not join the local gang, MS-13. Concerned for their lives, Antonio and his mother put their only belongings in one bag and began their migration North to the United States. Antonio and his mother's 2-month-long journey included riding on the *tren de la muerte* (train of death) also known as *la bestia* (the beast). They endured 3 days of hunger, and his mother was sexually assaulted as Antonio was held back by gang members on the train. Antonio's mother also sustained a broken arm during their migration. Upon arrival in Northern Mexico, they sought asylum on the border with the United States. Antonio was separated from his mother; his mother was detained and taken to an adult immigration detention center in Port Isabel, Texas, and Antonio was placed in a shelter for unaccompanied minors. After days at the shelter, Antonio was noncommunicative, withdrawn, soiling himself, and not eating or sleeping. At night, he was observed mumbling to himself and rocking back and forth. Shelter staff subsequently sought a psychological evaluation for developmental concerns.

Psychologists encounter clients from different developmental phases and an array of cultural backgrounds. Deciding how to approach the clinical interview and selecting specific measures to use, if any, may be an arduous task given the complexity of symptoms, language barriers, and the client's culture of origin. Nonetheless, a psychological evaluation is a medical necessity and warranted in cases like Antonio's. In this case, a *cultural clinical interview* emphasizing biopsychosocial factors is a priority. The biopsychosocial approach includes biological, psychological, and social factors and their complex interactions in understanding health. This model provides a holistic approach to the psychological assessment of culturally diverse populations.

The clinical interview is a vital component of the assessment process in every client, but it is even more important with culturally diverse groups and individuals like Antonio. In addition to basic clinical interviewing techniques, such as active and empathetic listening, issues of attitude and language must be navigated as well. How to navigate the language concerns and the use of interpreters will be covered in Chapter 6. Othmer and Othmer (2002) offer helpful strategies for enhancing rapport in the clinical interview, such as putting the client at ease, recognizing the client's emotional pain and showing compassion, displaying professionalism, and balancing multiple roles as a clinician. In addition to these basic clinical interviewing skills, we must consider other factors when assessing culturally diverse groups like Latinx people because the clinical interview will be a major source of information for determining if the client's experiences are pathological or culturally determined. Mental health clinicians will encounter clients like Antonio and many others from different parts of the world representing various cultures and beliefs. Thus, the cultural clinical interview is the most important component of the assessment process, and the psychotherapeutic skills used to build rapport, such as showing respect and authenticity via cultural humility, are critical.

It is best to avoid using a structured diagnostic clinical interview as the only clinical tool in a given assessment. Structured clinical interviews are based on DSM criteria which mainly capture psychopathology as it is experienced with dominant US culture, not cultures outside the United States. For example, in the case of Antonio, he was assessed in a clinical setting along the US–Mexico border, a place known as ground zero for the family separation crises imposed by US Customs and Border Patrol. As mentioned previously, recent research in this part of the country has revealed alarming rates of trauma (Mercado et al., 2019; Venta & Mercado, 2019). Children like Antonio and their families are fleeing trauma, poverty, and violence by migrating, and they risk their lives during migration. Many migrants continue to endure additional trauma during their migratory journey. Upon arrival to the United States, many children are separated from their families, as Antonio was, exposing them to additional trauma. In the case of Antonio, many of his mental health symptoms were ultimately judged to be related to posttraumatic distress. A structured clinical interview was not used. An unstructured approach highlighting the cultural context was critical in Antonio's evaluation. It is important to understand that mental health symptoms are expressed differently across cultural groups. Not everyone we encounter in clinical practice is going to meet specific diagnostic criteria included in the DSM.

Useful in many clinical circumstances, a structured clinical interview like the Structured Clinical Interview for the DSM-5 (SCID-5), covers a wide range of mental health concerns in the DSM-5, and two SCID-5 versions exist for personality disorders (American Psychiatric Association Publishing, 2019). For children, the Schedule for Affective Disorders and Schizophrenia for School-Age Children (K-SADs) Spanish version has been shown to have good psychometric properties with Spanish populations (Galicia-Moreno et al., 2018). In addition, semi-structured clinical interviews also exist that are more diagnostic-specific, like the Yale-Brown Obsessive Compulsive Scale (Y-BOCS) (Goodman et al., 1989), a measurement for obsessive compulsive disorder (OCD). A structured clinical interview like the SCID-5 includes pre-established items that a clinician should ask during the clinical interview. It can be a quite lengthy process to administer a structured interview, and a scoring criterion for each response is used to determine diagnostic criteria support across clinical disorder categories. Given that most structured clinical interviews are based on the DSM diagnostic algorithms and criteria, it should not be the first assessment tool used with culturally diverse groups especially in cases like Antonio's. In addition, an important consideration when using available assessment tools is to consider its psychometric properties, as discussed in Chapter 4. Shankman and colleagues (2018) found the SCID-5 to have substantial validity and reliability in a sample that included 22.6% of participants from Latinx descent; however, the study failed to identify specific background information of participants, including acculturation and language. Another recent study also noted the SCID-5, Clinician Version, as having excellent reliability, but no specific cultural background information of participants was identified (Osorio et al., 2019), thus presenting significant limitations. Although the SCID-5 appears to be a reliable measure to assess symptom severity regarding current and lifetime psychopathology in some Latinx groups, it is not considered the best clinical assessment to guide a diagnostic formulation with ethnic minority populations, especially those who have recently immigrated.

Other important sources of information to include in an initial assessment are behavioral rating scales like the Child Behavior Checklist (Achenbach, 1999), collateral information, and any pertinent documents (such as medical records which at times include a medication list and/or diagnosis from previous doctors). Family and caregivers can be an important source of information in the evaluation process given the role of *familismo* as a core Latinx cultural value. Emphasizing this cultural value in the assessment process will provide clinicians additional critical information that more likely would be ignored if using more traditional information-gathering approaches. There will be times where caregivers or family members will not be available, as in Antonio's case, who was separated from his mother. In these cases, it is the clinician's responsibility to get in contact with collateral reporters as much as possible. Many times, the psychologist has access to government employees or group home shelter staff who may have parent contact information or be able to provide collateral information themselves. However, there are times when no parental and background information is available. These are the most difficult cases, given that no developmental information is obtained.

Thus, relying on program/shelter staff is imperative, and other available resources are critical. Diagnoses may need to be made provisionally given the absence of developmental information. When family members can be contacted, cultural humility will assist in the clinical interview and will facilitate the collection of critical information needed for a holistic psychological evaluation of the client.

Using a cultural clinical interview approach, which is a combination of a semi-structured clinical interview with a core focus on the client's culture and background, will assist in providing additional critical and clinically sound information for a solid case conceptualization and a possible diagnostic formulation. Dr. Cervando Martinez (2013) emphasizes the importance of conducting a cross-cultural clinical interview and describes three basic elements in becoming a good interviewer: attaining a constant attitude of care, having empathy, and having compassion for those to whom we provide mental healthcare. Determining why the client was referred for a psychological evaluation and identifying the client's preferred language are foundational components of an effective clinical interview. Not always will a psychologist speak the same language as the client, and, at times, interpreters and translators may not be available. Using third parties can create a barrier to rapport-building and understanding the context of the client's story, symptoms, and behaviors. Speaking the same language as the client is preferred and is the most effective way of facilitating an effective clinical interview. If this is not possible, following and considering ethical guidelines is important, as many clients from diverse cultural backgrounds report their symptoms in different terms and may report mental health symptoms via physical complaints, something that is common in Latinx groups. Understanding and self-translating clinical language can be an arduous task. This is already a difficulty process but can even be more taxing with cross-cultural clients due to the need to navigate across languages, cultural, and social boundaries. Additional obstacles with interpreters and translators may arise, as covered in Chapter 6.

CULTURAL VALUES AND THE CLINICAL INTERVIEW

Incorporating Latinx cultural values in the clinical interview is essential, as discussed previously. Having and expressing an awareness of Latinx cultural values in the assessment process is important. For example, making effective use of *respeto*, *sympatia*, and *personalismo* during the assessment as guidance for interpersonal interactions with the client is recommended. Being respectful and personable is an important way to begin the therapeutic relationship. Doing so can be as simple as asking language preference and referring to the client as *usted* (when speaking in Spanish; Gonzalez-Prendes, Hindo, & Pardo, 2011). Also, engaging in *platica* (small talk) before the session begins and engaging in appropriate self-disclosure can be an example of expressing *personalismo* and *sympatia* (Edwards & Cardemil, 2015). In fact, it is common for a Latinx client to ask personal questions about the clinician's background, family, country of origin, and even immigration history. These questions should not necessarily be interpreted as efforts to push boundaries or seek too much information for ulterior motives, but rather to connect with the clinician.

Therefore, the information collected on the client's adherence of cultural values, whether collected via the cultural clinical interview or through other means, can provide insight into potential treatment strategies and interventions and possibly assist with treatment engagement. For instance, clients who endorse familistic values may benefit from interventions that may include family members; they may be encouraged to bring family members to sessions, something that is strongly recommended for those clients that do hold high levels of *familismo*. Similarly, when religion and spirituality are prominent values, incorporating these factors into treatment interventions is strongly recommended, as discussed previously. Moreover, a comprehensive awareness of the adherence of Latinx cultural values in a multigenerational family can assist the clinician in navigating the assessment process (Edwards & Cardemil, 2015). Thus, highlighting Latinx cultural values in the assessment process will aid in the selection of appropriate treatment strategies and interventions in addition to assisting in the conceptualization process. Pieterse and Miller (2009) postulated that "the role of the clinician cannot be overemphasized, as the clinician is the instrument through which a culturally inclusive assessment is undertaken" (p. 662).

As discussed previously, being well-versed in and understanding the clients' cultural background and having cultural humility will significantly assist the psychological assessment process with Latinx clients. In other words, clinicians must examine their own inner states, such as bias, tensions, preoccupations, and worries that may affect their perceptions and responses to the person they are trying to assist. If these personal aspects are not explored and examined, a clinician may do more harm than good in their attempt to assist a client. As mentioned previously, cultural humility is critical in the evaluation process and is even integrated in ethical codes of conduct for mental health professionals (National Association of Social Work, 2021). Recent political events and the recent political climate in the United States regarding immigration is one example of how current events may produce a climate of political divide that may affect adequate assessment of culturally diverse groups. If one's personal and political views carry an anti-immigration stance, a clinician may need to re-examine their role in working with immigrant clients and instead refer to other professionals who routinely work with this population. The same is true if a clinician appears to be more of an advocate than a psychologist when assessing a person of an immigrant or refugee background. For example, this type of bias in assessment can hinder clinical judgment in the evaluation process. Cultural humility in clinical interviewing is essential because, without it, we run the risk of compromising the psychological evaluation of clients from diverse cultural backgrounds, including Latinx persons.

To further understand the Latinx culture, specifically the Latinx client in the assessment room, it is important to understand the language and terminology commonly used when describing symptoms of mental health. For example, when conducting a clinical interview with a client of Latinx heritage, clients may mention terms including *nervios* or one of its derivatives, *nervioso, nerviosa, nerviosmo*.

Additionally, when referring to known cultural syndromes, such as *ataque de nervios*, clients may use the general term more loosely describing anxiety. The term *ansiedad* is also used, therefore it is important that the clinician conducting the clinical interview clarify what that term means to the client. *Ansiedad* may be a free-standing emotion or the result of an experience or event. It is also important to understand that some Latinx groups are very emotional beings, meaning that they use emotions to communicate in their everyday lives. Some clients may communicate with high energy and motivation and, in those cases, their actions may resemble manic-like symptoms. Clients may communicate with their hands and gestures, and some Latinx persons may even greet clinicians with a kiss on the cheek or a hug. These experiences should be explored in supervision in order to better understand the client and the meaning behind these exhibits of affection and respect.

PSYCHOPATHOLOGY VERSUS CULTURALLY SANCTIONED EXPERIENCES

Latinx persons may also describe symptoms that parallel mild psychotic symptoms (Lewis-Fernandez et al., 2009). For instance, some Latinx people report hearing their names being called, hearing whispers or other transient auditory phenomena, or seeing shadows, especially in the side of the visual field. These experiences may be a result of distress, trauma, lack of sleep, or other factors and do not necessarily indicate psychotic symptomology or related clinical diagnosis. These symptoms are commonly reported in the immigrant and refugee population as well. For example, we assessed a client who was referred for evaluation to rule out a psychotic disorder. He was separated from his father at the US–Mexico border and sent to a shelter for unaccompanied minors, even though he entered the United States with his caregiver. Program staff were concerned because of the odd behaviors he was exhibiting. For example, the client was fidgety, pacing back and forth in his room, observed talking to himself, and reported "seeing shadows" at night. Concerned for his health and safety, program staff decided to seek a psychological evaluation before referring the client to a psychiatrist for possible medication management for psychotic symptoms. Via a cultural humility approach, a cultural clinical interview assisted in ruling out a psychotic presentation. During the assessment, it was discovered that the teenage boys' symptoms and odd behaviors were instead acute stress and trauma symptoms. The "shadow" he saw was only visible at night and occurred in the context of significant anxiety and distress. When program staff observed that he was "responding to internal stimuli," the teenage boy was praying to his ancestors to be reunited with his father. Indeed, religious beliefs are important to probe in the assessment process with culturally diverse groups (Weinstein & Jimenez, 2021). There are times when religious beliefs and behavior may seem extreme or even pathological to a mental health professional. Among some culturally diverse groups, including some Latinx persons, rigidly held religious views are common and are not in and of themselves pathological. Some clients may even share personal religious experiences, such as contact with a divine presence that markedly affected them and even changed their lives. These experiences may be puzzling to some clinicians who do not share the same religious beliefs. However, cultural humility would appropriately guide the clinician and reduce the risk of rendering a misdiagnosis based on culturally bound religious experiences and beliefs. Furthermore, without cultural humility, a clinician may even ignore an important core resiliency factor that may aid in abating symptoms of mental health and distress.

The clinical interview in the psychological assessment process strives to elicit, observe, and note the client's symptoms of psychopathology and personal customs while simultaneously placing these in a social and cultural context determined by the person's background. Psychopathology is affected by cultural and social factors; therefore, these factors should not be ignored. Mezzich, Caracci, Fabrega, and Kirmayer (2009) emphasize that the process of evaluating whether something is cultural versus pathological is done during a "stepping-back process" and is part of cultural formulation. Dr. Freddy Paniagua (Dana, 2013) notes that there are important difficulties in establishing a distinction between psychopathological conditions in culturally diverse groups, such as limited time in sessions with minority groups due to attrition, Medicaid, and insurance barriers. However, he stresses using the guidelines suggested previously and that he believes are crucial in assisting the differential diagnosis process and helping practitioners in making the critical distinction between pathology and culture in clinical practice. For example, the following three guidelines are suggested:

1. Consultation with relatives and including folk healers, *curanderos*, to assist mental health professionals in the recognition of symptoms.
2. Clinicians' self-assessment of biases and prejudice that may impact diagnosis and treatment of culturally diverse client.
3. Being culturally appropriate when questioning to encourage the client and family members to report about culture-related situations they believe could explain the origin of symptoms.

These guidelines are important when working with Latinx clients in clinical settings. The first highlights the importance of including the family and, when needed, consulting folk healers. A good folk-healer will also share the importance of seeing a mental health professional. During my career with different Latinx groups on the West Coast, East Coast, and the South, I have met various *curanderos* (folk-healers) who were part of interdisciplinary team meetings. If a client believes in this spiritual practice, it is important to respect and include this belief and practice in the assessment process. I have met *curanderos* who are very astute and understand the importance of mental health evaluations and treatment. I have found that working alongside them and respecting/accepting the client's beliefs furthers the assessment and evaluation process and assists with treatment engagement (Turner et al., 2016). However, it is important to know the trusted and reliable *curanderos* in your communities, as there are a few who may exploit clients and their families. The second and third guidelines encompass some of the characteristics of cultural humility in clinical interviewing that we described earlier.

Due to the recent political climate in the United States, it is pivotal to also include sociopolitical context in the cultural clinical interview. The clinical interview should cover a social-ecological framework (Bronfenbrenner, 1992) that includes the dynamics surrounding documented and undocumented status in the immediate family and friends and that includes familial-related stress. Once rapport has been established, reviewing clients' immigration status and its role in familial dynamics is important and will arise naturally. Thus, these additional three guidelines are critical to include in a culturally sound clinical interview once rapport has been established:

1. Facilitating a social-ecological framework in the interview is critical to include the client's experience and the contextual risk and protective factors that may distract from or further healthy adaptation.
2. Once language and level of acculturation has been assessed, the psychologist will determine what specific cognitive and personal measures will be facilitated if needed for the psychological evaluation. There will be times that psychological testing will not be needed if a thorough cultural clinical interview is facilitated.
3. Clinicians are encouraged to select instruments that have demonstrated measurement equivalence and to consider the cultural loading and linguistic demands of instruments prior to inclusion in their evidence-based assessment batteries. (This is discussed in Chapter 4.)

CULTURE-BOUND SYNDROMES AMONG LATINX PERSONS

As we have discussed, in the psychological assessment of Latinx people, it is vital to understand the role of culture in order to prevent and/or minimize overdiagnosing, underdiagnosing, or misdiagnosing psychopathologies. *Cultural-bound syndromes* were first introduced in the DSM-IV and described as "25 forms of aberrant behavior that are referred as locality specific troubling experiences that are limited to certain societies or cultural areas." The text discussed cultural variables across several disorders. For example, Latinx persons listed four symptoms including *ataque de nervios*, described as an out-of-conscious state resulting from evil spirts. The symptoms include crying, trembling, verbal or physical aggression, and intense heat in the chest, and many times are associated with stressful events (e.g., death of a loved one, divorce or separation, or witnessing an accident including a family member). *Colera* is a syndrome in which anger and rage disturb body balances, leading to headache, screaming, stomach pain, loss of consciousness, and fatigue. The third syndrome, called *mal de ojo* or *ojo*, occurs when medical symptoms such as vomiting, fever, diarrhea, mental health problems (anxiety, depression), or other unexplained medical illness result from the *evil eye* cast by another person. This is commonly reported in infants and children, although adults may experience this as well. To prevent *ojo*, many families wear a red bracelet or a bracelet with an eye-shaped charm or various saint emblems. The fourth culture-bound syndrome illustrated in the DSM-IV-TR is *susto*, which is tiredness and weakness resulting from a frightening and startling experience and may sometimes bring appetite and sleep disturbances. The DSM-5 replaced the notion of culture-bound syndromes with (1) *cultural syndromes*, or "clusters of symptoms and attributions that tend to co-occur among individuals in specific cultural groups, communities, or contexts . . . that are recognized locally as coherent patterns of experience" (p. 758); (2) *cultural idioms of distress*, or "ways of expressing distress that may not involve specific symptoms or syndromes, but that provide collective, shared ways of experiencing and talking about personal or social concerns" (p. 758); and (3) *cultural explanations of distress or perceived causes*, "labels, attributions, or features of an explanatory model that indicate culturally recognized meaning or etiology for symptoms, illness, or distress" (p. 758). The DSM-5 made a timely improvement, as mentioned previously, by including an Emerging Measures Section III to include the Cultural Formulation Interview (CFI) and the World Health Organization Disability Assessment Schedule 2.0 (WHODAS) measures. Rather than a simple list of culture-bound syndromes, the DSM-5 updated the cross-cultural variations in presentations to included cultural concepts of distress, thus aiding in the clinical utility of the DSM-5 and including a clinical interview tool.

CONCLUSION

The culture clinical interview is enhanced by the clinician's cultural humility. As discussed previously, the cultural formulation requires the mental health clinician to be aware of the cultural identity of the client, cultural explanations the client may have about his or her symptoms/illness, and cultural factors related to the client's functioning (APA, 2013). In addition, being aware of the differences between the clinician and the individual with respect to social class and culture is important. A cultural clinical interview will aid in an effective case formulation. This chapter also expands on existing guidelines when working with Latinx clients in the clinical setting.

4

Psychometric Issues in Assessment with Latinx Persons

OVERVIEW

The American Psychological Association (APA) Ethics Code (Standard 9.02 Use of Assessments; APA, 2010) states that assessment instruments need to be validated and reliable for use with individuals of the populations tested. In the event that no such instruments exist, the professional is instructed to "describe the strengths and limitations of test results and interpretation" (Standard 9.02). The same standard indicates that psychologists should use methods that are appropriate to the client's language preference and competence. Additionally, individual characteristics, such as test-taking abilities and cultural differences, must be considered (Standard 9.06, Interpreting Assessment Results). When working effectively with Latinx persons in the United States, then, it is likely that cultural and linguistic factors will need to be considered in the assessment context. These challenges and the APA's ethics code underlie the three major topics in reviewed in this chapter. First, we briefly review background data across disciplines that suggest that language and cultural factors can indeed affect testing results. Second, we introduce the Culture Language Interpretive Matrix (Flanagan, Ortiz, & Alfonso, 2013). Third, we discuss the matter of cross-cultural psychometrics, reviewing Pina, Gonzales, Holly, Zerr, and Wynne's (2013) approach to evidence-based assessment with ethnic minorities and utilizing examples from commonly used instruments.

EFFECTS OF LANGUAGE AND CULTURE ON PSYCHOLOGICAL ASSESSMENT

In this chapter, we build on a recent systematic review conducted by members of our research team (Bailey, Venta, & Langley, 2019) in order to underscore the basic premise that language and cultural factors affect psychological assessments. Fundamentally, a wide array of research from varied disciplines indicates that completing assessment tasks using a non-native language can be detrimental to someone's performance (Kisser et al., 2012; Sotelo-Dynega et al., 2013)—a serious concern when testing Latinx persons (21% of the US population speaks Spanish; US Census Bureau, 2015; 2018). The review by Bailey et al. (2019) concluded that Spanish-English bilinguals are generally at a disadvantage on measures of verbal ability across the lifespan and, perhaps relatedly, on instruments used to test individuals for placement in special education or gifted and talented programs; however, they display advantages on tasks of metalinguistic awareness, statistical learning, theory of mind development, and some areas of effortful control. Importantly, discrepancies between bilinguals and monolinguals on psychological assessments like these are not resolved by testing in both languages (Gross, Buac, & Kaushanskaya, 2014), leading for calls to provide different norms for psychological tests based on subcategories of bilingualism (Bailey et al., 2019).

The aforementioned biases in testing data from bilingual individuals is likely to be even more pronounced in instruments that are less standardized and more reliant on self-disclosure, including clinical interviews. Indeed, the effects of language on performance are exacerbated when the tasks require subtle complexity, like use of metaphors, jokes, or sarcasm (Dunnigan, McNall, & Mortimer, 1993; Homayounpour & Movahedi, 2012; McNamara, 1997). These difficulties can prompt feelings of being misunderstood in a clinical context (Homayounpour & Movahedi, 2012). Moreover, assessment in a second language can influence the content that is disclosed and how it is described: memories may be better and more accurately recalled in the client's native language rather than in a second language (Kinginger, 2004; Pavlenko, 2006); native language processing may be deeper and more syntactically detailed (see review by Clahsen & Felser, 2006); describing an event using the same language that was used at the time of the event can result in a narrative that is more emotionally and expressively rich (Javier, Barroso & Muñoz, 1993); and clients may experience more physiological arousal and differences in brain activity in response to emotionally laden words in their first rather than second language (Harris, 2004; Harris, Ayçiçeği, & Gleason, 2003; Hsu, Jacobs, & Conrad, 2015).

For all of these reasons, the Council of National Psychological Associations for the Advancement of Ethnic Minority Interests, in their monograph *Testing and Assessment with Persons & Communities of Color*, recommends that providers strive for the following (Reynaga-Abiko et al., 2016, p. 27):

1. In addition to the required training and experience in psychological assessment, ensure formal training in the assessment of Latina/os, including understanding of Latina/o-specific cultural constructs (Acevedo-Polakovich et al., 2007).

2. Maintain working knowledge about the specific Latina/o group(s) with which an assessment is being conducted (Dana, 1998).

3. Use only properly normed, standardized, and translated measures chosen specifically based on the Latina/o client's ethnic subgroup, acculturation level, language proficiency, education level, socioeconomic status, and other relevant demographic factors (Reynaga-Abiko, 2005).

4. Assess the language abilities and fluency of the Latina/o client to determine the most appropriate assessment instrument(s), using interpreters
as necessary (Acevedo-Polakovich et al., 2007).

5. Interpret and report assessment results in a culturally contextualized
manner (Acevedo-Polakovich et al., 2007; Alamilla & Wojcik, 2013), including family and/or community members in the feedback session(s) when
appropriate (Reynaga-Abiko, 2005).

6. Consult with an expert in Latina/o assessment whenever needed to
ensure cultural competence throughout the assessment process (i.e., from
instrument choice to interpretation and report writing; Acevedo-Polakovich
et al., 2007).

While the first, second, fifth, and sixth recommendations may be facilitated by
reviewing the content provided in Chapters 1, 2, 3, and 6 of this book, the third
and fourth will be addressed directly in the remainder of this chapter and in
Chapter 5.

THE CULTURE-LANGUAGE INTERPRETIVE MATRIX

All of the studies just described indicate that there are potential problems of ad-
vantage/disadvantage in psychological testing with bilingual individuals and that
these difficulties may also be present—and perhaps even pronounced—in tasks
that are more reliant upon self-disclosure, like clinical interview. While determining in which language to conduct a psychological assessment is a complex
area of empirical research on its own (see the Multidimensional Assessment
Model for Bilingual Individuals by Ochoa & Ortiz, 2005, for instance), research
has also established that linguistic dominance is not the only factor at play in
testing because it interacts with cultural loading in relation to test validity issues
(e.g., Rhodes, Ochoa, & Ortiz, 2005).

The Culture-Language Test Classification system (Flanagan et al., 2007;
Flanagan & Ortiz, 2001; McGrew & Flanagan, 1998) was developed to address
the question of whether low cognitive or achievement test scores reflect cultural/
linguistic differences or disorder (i.e., "difference versus disorder"; Ortiz, Ochoa,
& Dynda, 2012). Specifically, existing norm-referenced tests were categorized
according to their hypothesized cultural loading (based on bilingual examinee performance) on the Culture-Language Test Classifications Matrix and on
its successor, the Culture-Language Interpretive Matrix. The Culture-Language
Interpretive Matrix arranges psychological assessments across axes representing
linguistic demand and cultural loading based on mean score differences between
English-language learners and English speakers as well as expert review (Styck
& Watkins, 2014). For example, a fluid reasoning task like Matrix Reasoning
on the Wechsler Intelligence Scale for Children is reported to have low cultural
loading and a low degree of linguistic demand, whereas a subtest like Vocabulary
or Comprehension is considered to have high cultural loading and linguistic

demand. Client performance is hypothesized to be least affected when both cultural loading and linguistic demand are low and, conversely, most affected when both are high.

Individuals seeking to use the Culture-Language Interpretive Matrix could purchase the broader cross-battery software in order to do so (Flanagan, Ortiz, & Alfonso, 2017). The Matrix first asks a clinician to make a clinical judgment about their client's "degree of difference" in terms of acculturative learning and language experience compared to the normative base for the instrument. The clinician then proceeds to enter their test results in the software, which provides interpretive results regarding the hypothesized effects of language and culture on test performance by arranging results in tiers from level 1 (lowest in cultural loading/linguistic demand) to 5 (highest in cultural loading/linguistic demand). If a client's test scores decline from tiers 1 to tier 5, the profile suggests bias and lack of validity. Sample interpretive statements are provided indicating that, for example, when results are hypothesized to have been highly impacted by cultural/ linguistic variables they should be considered invalid for the purposes of psychological testing.

While the Culture-Language Interpretive Matrix has been influential in, first, arranging existing tools along two dimensions that are important to working with Latinx persons and well-covered in this book (i.e., acculturation/cultural values and language), and second, readily including linguistic and cultural concerns in the overall validity of testing data, it has not been without its criticisms. Indeed, concerns remain regarding how experts were selected for the arrangement of tests on the matrix and also for how consensus among experts was attained (Styck & Watkins, 2014). Furthermore, emerging empirical evidence stands in contrast to the basic premise of the Culture-Language Interpretive Matrix. Work by Kranzler and colleagues (2010), for instance, indicated that most known English-language learner students in their sample did not follow the pattern of decline hypothesized by the Matrix. Similarly, Styck and Watkins (2014) noted that only 11% of English-language learner students who were referred for testing to determine eligibility for special education services followed the hypothesized profile. Styck and Watkins (2014) as well as Meyer (2013) and Van Deth (2013) found that the Matrix profile could not discriminate between English-language learner students and English-speaker students. In all of the aforementioned studies, widely used standardized assessment instruments were utilized (i.e., Woodcock-Johnson, Weschler, Kaufman). In sum, the Culture-Language Interpretive Matrix has made meaningful theoretical contributions that may be useful for a clinician working with Latinx persons in the United States, but it requires further empirical testing.

CROSS-CULTURAL PSYCHOMETRICS

In the absence of an empirically based standard procedure for determining the effect of linguistic and cultural factors on testing data, clinicians working with

Latinx persons in the United States find themselves making test selections inde-
pendently. In doing so, we hope that the cross-cultural psychometric properties of
a given test is considered. In this chapter, we focus on understanding the psychometric properties that may be particularly useful in this application, and we provide examples of these properties. Overall, these topics go beyond the calculation
of basic psychometric properties like internal consistency or validity to examine
whether psychometric properties are consistent across meaningful population
subgroups (e.g., cultural groups or immigrant groups)—considerations cited in
the *Standards for Educational and Psychological Testing* (AERA, APA, & NCME,
1999) and in the American Psychological Association's *Handbook of Clinical
Psychology* (Norcross, VandenBos, & Freedheim, 2016). We structure this chapter
around Pina, Gonzales, Holly, Zerr, and Wynne's (2013) evidence-based clinical
assessment of ethnic minority youth, although the same psychometric principles
are applicable to adult clients. In doing so, we discuss the two major features of
Pina et al's (2013) review: measurement equivalence and method bias.

Measurement equivalence includes both *item equivalence* (which can include
configural, metric, threshold, and item uniqueness invariance) and *construct
validity equivalence* (which includes functional and scalar equivalence; Hui &
Triandis, 1985; Knight et al., 2002; Pina et al., 2013). Broadly, configural invariance asks whether an assessment instrument demonstrates the same factor structure across groups (Ghorpade, Hattrup, & Lackritz, 1999; Millsap & Yun-Tein,
2004; Pina et al., 2013; Vandenberg & Lance, 2000). If the configural invariance
of an instrument is low, some items from that instrument do not load onto their
hypothesized (and previously documented factor) when the scale is completed
in a different cultural group. On the other hand, evidence of the same factor
structure across cultural groups would indicate that the groups share the same
concept of whatever construct is being measured. For example, a recent study of
the Beck Depression Inventory II in inpatient adolescents found the posited two-
factor structure of the instrument (cognitive-affective and somatic) in African
American/Black, Caucasian/White, and Hispanic/Latinx adolescents, suggesting
that the three groups have the same concept of depression.

Pina and colleagues (2013) are careful to note that evidence of configural invariance is insufficient to support the use of an instrument across groups, citing
that *metric invariance*—the extent to which the meaning of individual assessment
items differs across groups (Labouvie & Ruetsch, 1995; Pina et al., 2013; Raykov,
2004)—may be a greater clinical consideration. Indeed, Pina and colleagues (2013)
note that culturally embedded terms like "*nervios*" in Spanish may be mistaken
for less-culturally laden terms, like the more general "nervous," thereby leading to
different interpretations of an item across groups. Similarly, items intended to assess depression by probing feelings of "punishment" may not perform equivalently
in cultural groups where religious notions of punishment are common (Azocar
et al., 2001). In our work, we have speculated that an item from the Child PTSD
Symptom Scale (Foa et al., 2001) may have similar problems in Spanish-speaking
youth. The item, which is intended to measure hypervigilance in a posttraumatic
reaction, reads, "has *estado demasiado cuidadoso(a) y atento(a)*" which includes

positively valenced concepts like being careful and attentive, rather than negatively valenced concepts like being hypervigilant (Venta & Mercado, 2019).

Finally, *threshold invariance* (Pina et al., 2013; Widaman & Reise, 1997) asks how severely a construct must be experienced before the client endorses a given item, and *item uniqueness invariance* (Byrne, Shavelson, & Muthén, 1989; Pina et al., 2013) refers to the unexplained variance in item endorsement. Ideally, assessment instruments would be subjected to empirical analyses of configural, metric, threshold, and item uniqueness invariance in an effort to establish item equivalence between the group in which the measure was developed and the ethnic, racial, gender groups to which the client belongs.

In order to fully evaluate measurement equivalence, empirical work should also endeavor to examine *construct validity equivalence*—the notion that "the construct being assessed has similar precursors, consequences, and/or correlates across groups" (Pina et al., 2013). Specifically, *functional equivalence* assesses whether the slopes of construct validity relations are consistent across groups, whereas *scalar equivalence* evaluates the intercepts of those relations (Knight & Hill, 1998; Knight et al., 2002). An assessment instrument should have demonstrated both construct validity equivalence and item equivalence with respect to the client's cultural, ethnic, or racial group before being included in an evidence-based assessment. For example, in assessing a self-report of victimization and exclusion among Latinx and European American adolescents, Buhs, McGinley, and Toland (2010) demonstrated that, across ethnic groups, links between the instrument in question and related variables like internalizing, demographics, and peer nominations were similar. Pina, Little, Knight, and Silverman (2009) undertook a similar study linking the Revised Children's Manifest Anxiety Scale and theoretically related measures of fear and depression in White and Latinx children.

A final consideration noted by Pina and colleagues (2013) centers on *method bias*—the notion that assessment methods like interviews or questionnaires produce nonequivalent data across groups (e.g., Van de Vijver & Leung, 2011). For instance, Asian American ratings of social anxiety are significantly higher than those of European Americans on questionnaire-based measures but significantly lower on interview-based measures, suggesting method bias in the assessment of social anxiety (Matsumoto & Kupperbusch, 2001). Attention to method variance introduces a number of other assessment considerations related to the language of assessment that were previously discussed.

CONCLUSION

Clinicians are encouraged to select instruments that have demonstrated measurement equivalence and to consider the cultural loading and linguistic demands of instruments prior to inclusion in their evidence-based assessment batteries. Much of the next chapter will focus on the properties of specific tests for use with Latinx persons. Still, existing literature often assumes homogeneity across ethnic groups, with little consideration for the critical variables (e.g., cultural values, norms, language, etc.) reviewed in the Introduction and Chapters 1–3. Moreover, measurement equivalence and method bias studies are limited, partly because they require substantial resources and pose unique methodological challenges (Fernandez, Boccaccini, & Noland, 2007). Clinicians may find the four-step approach put forth by Fernandez, Boccaccini, and Noland (2007) helpful. First, clinicians identify tests available in their language of interest; second, available research must be reviewed so that; third, research can be reviewed for its applicability to the specific client; and, finally, the clinician can make an overall determination about the level of research support for using the selected test with an identified client. Though the four-step approach was originally devised for clinicians seeking to identify and select translated tests, it is based on the professional testing standards put forth by the *Standards for Educational and Psychological Testing* (AERA, APA, & NCME, 1999), which addresses "fairness in testing" more generally and may therefore be useful to clinicians working with immigrant populations.

Instruments for Psychological Assessment with Latinx Persons

OVERVIEW

This chapter focuses on the careful selection of psychological batteries that include cognitive and personality measures. As mentioned in the previous chapter, there will be times when psychological testing will not be needed once a thorough cultural clinical interview is conducted. However, when psychological testing is a critical component of the referral at hand, it is then crucial that careful selection of measures be assured.

IMPORTANCE OF CAREFUL MEASURE SELECTION

In the field of clinical psychology, there are many psychological instruments available, including cognitive and personality measures, that psychologists can choose from. As highlighted in previous chapters, psychologists must consider the psychometric properties and standardization sample of published instruments in deciding appropriate fit for the culturally diverse client. It is the responsibility of the psychologist to take into consideration racial, ethnic, and linguistic differences between the client and the standardization sample and to determine how culture and language might affect the administration, interpretation, and overall psychological assessment process. Cognitive and personality measures include instruments and batteries that are only a part of the overall holistic evaluation process of the person, and these should be supplemented with proper clinical interviewing, as described in Chapter 3.

Researching best practices for working with Latinx people, including immigrant groups, in research and clinical setting is important (Mercado, Venta, & Irizarry, 2019). Mercado and colleagues (2019) highlight the need for further examination of specific assessments used in the clinical settings with Latinx clients to include psychometric and linguistic considerations and the importance of having realistic solutions. This book has identified prior guidelines and expanded newer guidelines to facilitate best practices when working with Latinx groups in the psychological assessment setting. Upon completion of a sound cultural clinical interview as discussed previously, once the level of acculturation has been assessed during the clinical interview and degree of language preference has been determined, the clinician will determine which specific cognitive and personal measures will be appropriate. Once this is determined, the next step is for the clinician to select instruments that have demonstrated measurement equivalence across ethnic, racial, and cultural subgroups and to consider the cultural loading and linguistic demands of instruments prior to inclusion in their evidence-based assessment batteries.

In addition to using appropriate standardized measures, it is critical for clinicians to use multiple sources of information when treating and assessing Latinx clients to minimize errors in assessment. Obtaining a cultural clinical interview that includes comprehensive psychosocial history and a mental health status examination will not be enough in many cases, and the use of multiple sources of information is critical. For example, collecting collateral information including a family interview and an environmental risk assessment, along with any other relevant information is important. Clinicians must be cautious when interpreting the assessment results of culturally diverse clients to avoid over- or underpathologizing. The unbiased interpretation of assessment results for the Latinx client and those of culturally diverse backgrounds may be possible only when the clinician is knowledgeable and sensitive to multicultural issues and using culturally appropriate assessment measures (Kouyoumdjian, Zamboanga, & Hansen, 2003).

Nonetheless, there are many challenges when attempting to effectively assess Latinx patients using psychological instruments, as previously noted. It is likely that bias can occur at various levels of the testing process: at the level of items or scales or during the interview, administration, and interpretation of findings. Throughout history, norms for most available psychological batteries include low levels of representation of Latinx persons, and most do not include socioeconomic status, immigration, language fluency, or acculturation information. Moreover, psychological instruments may probe for symptom expression that differs from how Latinx people define psychopathology, experience symptoms, and describe experiences. Therefore, the clinician must be cautious when using the norms and interpretive data from conventional measures due to their Eurocentric assumptions (Dana, 1998). As discussed in previous chapters, an array of factors are crucial to the psychosocial functioning and mental health of Latinx people, and these should be incorporated into the assessment process: acculturation level, ethnic identity, language fluency, socioeconomic status (including education, occupation, and wealth), and religion/spirituality. The incorporation of these factors is consistent with published guidelines and cultural formulation models (American Psychiatric Association, 2017).

It is important to keep in mind that there is no specific method of psychological assessment recommended in this book because the method chosen must depend on the rationale, referral question, individual's history and context, and purpose of the assessment (Meyer et al., 2001). To provide more valid assessment of Latinx persons, assessment instruments can be adapted by translation, re-normed to include a representative sample of Latinx people, or replaced as new measures are created (Gutierrez, 2002). Also, there will be times when psychological instruments will not be needed, as discussed in previous chapters. However, in some clinical cases, psychological measures will aid in the evaluation process. When this is the case, we must further address and examine what specific variables need to be assessed. In other words, why was the client referred to you? Often, the abilities that need to be measured do not have cultural equivalence (Helms, 1992). For example, Puente and Perez-Garcia (2000) noted that time is an important variable in determining intelligence in North American cultures, and we must examine if time is even valuable in the client's cultural background if we are to confound it with intelligence. The authors also recommend utilizing measures that are adequately translated and have appropriate norms.

Differing degrees of English fluency and multilingualism among Latinx persons further complicate the selection of assessment instruments. For instance, if an assessment aims to determine the presence or absence of a specific learning disability in a bilingual client, consideration of fluency and, potentially, bilingual assessment are critical. Olvera and Gomez-Cervillo (2011) stress the importance of conducting a bilingual assessment when assessing for learning disorders, with one assessment conducted in the client's primary language and another in the secondary language by a qualified bilingual psychologist or a monolingual psychologist with a qualified interpreter. A qualified interpreter should also have firsthand knowledge of the client's culture because they must adequately interpret not only the content but also the emotionality of the language (Olvera & Gomez-Cervillo, 2011; Chapter 6 discusses suggestions when working with interpreters). Assessing the client in both their primary and second languages is recommended because learning disability is manifested in both languages. By administering both assessments, the assessment data will provide a clearer understanding of the client's strengths and weaknesses and support linguistically appropriate interventions that recognize the bilingual context of the client. In many cases, children learning English appear to have similar challenges as children who are suspected of having a learning disability (Diaz-Rico & Weed, 2006), and bilingual assessment is one way to distinguish the two groups.

As previously discussed, a significant concern surrounding the psychological assessment of Latinx persons is the use of potentially biased standardized instruments (Reynaga-Abiko et al., 2016). Most psychological measures have been developed in English and standardized using normative samples consisting of mainly European Americans and few, if any, Latinx people (Butcher et al., 2007). However, in recent years, the psychology field has witnessed important efforts toward ensuring fairness in the testing and assessment of Latinx persons

(Curiel et al., 2016). A number of measures have been either developed for or adapted/normed for Latinx and Spanish-speaking individuals. Similar efforts for equity are also present in other related mental health fields (Alegria, Nakash, & NeMoyer, 2018). This chapter provides an overview of some of the most commonly used and researched assessment instruments with Latinx and Spanish-speaking populations in the United States

Language is an important factor to consider during the test selection decision-making process. Spanish-speaking Latinx persons may share the same language yet represent diverse cultural and linguistic backgrounds. For instance, they may vary greatly along the lines on country of origin, sociopolitical, economic, educational experiences, and spiritual/religious. In addition, acculturation and use of Spanish in the family vary widely in Spanish-speaking families (Elliott, 2012). It is important to understand that these variables affect test-taking abilities and test scores. The Pruebas Publicadas en Espanol (PPE) (Assessments Published in Spanish) is one resource that is available to assist in the test selection process. It is a comprehensive bibliography of Spanish tests (e.g., academic, mental health). PPE provides information that includes the translation and adaption processes used as well as the appropriate existing norms and the availability of different test components in both Spanish and English. The information contained in PPE maybe used to compare tests across domains, thus furthering test selection (Carlos & Gonzalez, 20015). Regarding acculturation, López, Ehly, and García-Vásquez (2002), for instance, highlighted that when assessing intelligence with a Latinx client, is important to consider that incremental improvement in US school performance occurs as acculturation increases.

Additionally, as discussed in previous chapters, professionals must understand and report on the psychometric value of any assessment used. It is not always possible to choose assessments with psychometric support specifically for the youth or adult client's demographic. Many assessments have been standardized or utilized with psychometric vigor in other languages, but research is still lacking to support the use of common assessment measures and tests of intellectual abilities in immigrant populations. Furthermore, those with psychometric support often have "fine print" associated with their use. For example, the Woodcock-Muñoz Test of Cognitive Abilities and Achievement Test has only been validated for use with individuals who have been in the United States for less than 2 years (Schrank et al., 2005). Understanding the psychometric properties of and reporting caveats for each chosen measure and assessment's use will decrease the chance for invalid results or results that may be misconstrued. It is good practice to include a validity section in a psychological report in order to emphasize the strengths and weaknesses (from a validity standpoint) of the data collection and reporting process and truthfully acknowledge aspects of the evaluation process that call results into question. Psychological measures included in this section were selected from instruments' with psychometric properties considered acceptable with certain Latinx groups and on the strength of the authors' experience using these measures in clinical settings. It is recommended that clinicians review related instruments' psychometric properties and administration manuals for further test data.

COGNITIVE MEASURES

A multitude of variables must be considered when assessing the cognitive functioning of a Latinx client. As discussed previously, level of acculturation and language proficiency are two key factors to consider when assessing a Latinx client's cognitive functioning. The Latinx client's experiences in school, whether some or all of their education occurred in the United States, and the language of their schooling may be associated with test results and variables that affect cognitive abilities, such as exposure to new learning environments, novel intellectual stimulation, and positive changes in socioeconomic environment (Weiss, Prifitera, & Munoz, 2015). Formal education conveys cultural information and conventions for thinking and categorization skills, all of which may affect both verbal and nonverbal test performance. Customs concerning verbal communication may evolve through exposure to US culture and educational settings. For some immigrants, prior experiences with formal education may have been limited due to geographic constraints, economic barriers, or sociopolitical constraints affecting access to educational resources. Experience with test-taking in general and acquisition of test-taking skills will likely have a positive influence on the individual's performance on cognitive assessments. Experience with US educational culture is likely to facilitate the development of bilingual skills in native Spanish speakers, which may influence performance on cognitive tests. For example, bilingual children exhibit greater inhibitory control and executive functioning skills than has been observed in monolingual children (Bialystok, Craik, & Luk, 2008; Carlson & Meltzoff, 2008). Younger children acquiring English may take 5 to 7 years, on average, to approach grade-level in academic areas (Ramirez, 1991). Culture is a major factor in the psychological assessment and the selection process of psychological instruments. Prior concerns noted by Lopez and Romero (1988) in intellectual testing with Latinx clients included the use of interpreters, using performance scales only, attempting to take language into account when interpreting scores, and inappropriately relying on Spanish-speaking staff for instructions. The authors stressed that these procedures are inappropriate and some are unethical. In addition, relying on one instrument or administering an intellectual measure or nonverbal measure with a Spanish-speaking client who recently immigrated to the United States would also not be appropriate. Facilitating a cultural and holistic assessment is critical. Competent clinicians must be aware of the ethical and appropriate test procedures to follow when working with people of color, including Latinx persons. In addition, as previously discussed, level of acculturation is a crucial component of the assessment process in general, as is determining the client's country of origin, language proficiency and preference, education, and income, all of which may aid in the interpretation of cognitive testing data. Moreover, examining the psychometric properties, including cultural bias, of the test is important. Using tests with specific instructions and protocols is imperative. It is important to be cautious when using nonverbal cognitive measures because nonverbal tests are not necessarily non–culturally biased assessments (Puente & Perez-Garcia, 2000) because some yield differences in certain cultural groups (Mahurin, Espino, & Holifield, 1992). A few measures, on the other hand, have been found to have cultural equivalence (e.g., the Category test, which is a neuropsychological screening measure that evaluates abstract thinking; Cuevas & Osterich,1990).

Upon reviewing collateral information and pertinent records and assessing historical and current language of instruction, the psychologist should determine the primary academic skills language. For instance, if the client has received instruction in Spanish in their home country or in a bilingual program, then it is important to assess academic skills in Spanish and administer, for example, the Bateria III Woodcock Munoz: Prueba de Aprovechamiento (Muños-Sandoval, Woodcock, McGrew, & Mather, 2005). This assessment is best used by a psychologist who is fluent in Spanish or with the assistance of a qualified interpreter. It is important to note that the Batería III, similar to other Spanish assessments, was normed with Spanish-speaking populations typically not represented in the United States. Thus, the examiner is advised to take precautions in the interpretation of the data, and an evaluation report should include this caveat.

Historically, Latinx persons have underperformed on intelligence tests by about 15–20 points depending on the sample (Rhodes, Ochoa, & Ortiz, 2005). This lower performance has been attributed to issues of validity (Rhodes et al., 2005). Note that simplistic notions of test bias have led to simplistic methods of addressing it in testing. It is important for examiners to use a range of methods and procedures when evaluating intelligence and learning disability in Latinx populations, such as modifying tests, using nonverbal tests, using native language assessments, and testing in English without any modifications. *Testing of the limits* is one avenue for modifying aspects of the test procedures. This approach is an attempt to examine how the client would do if allowances were made for language differences, timing, or other factors. For instance, the examiner may continue to administer items after discontinuation rules have been met. Other modifications include repeating instructions, explaining task concepts prior to administration to enhance comprehension, or eliminating or modifying time constraints that inhibit the examinee's performance (Ortiz & Menlo, 2015). Although the examinee's performance may improve, the standardization procedures have been violated, thereby invalidating the profile. When this happens, the results become invalid, precluding normative comparisons and interpretation. It is important when testing of the limits is done that this is used as supplemental data and that a thorough explanation of the profile and the Testing of the limits is included. For similar reasons, the use of interpreters can also affect the validity of test results, even with a trained and qualified interpreter. These concerns are not new in the field of psychological testing. In fact, significant concerns in intellectual testing of children of color, in particular Latinx and African American children, were raised in the 1930s.

Dr. George I. Sanchez (1906–1972), a pioneer in Mexican American psychology and founder of Chicano Psychology movement, was the first to write on themes of Mexican American well-being. In his early work, he contributed four articles (between 1932 and 1934) discussing intelligence testing of Latinx children. In Dr. Sanchez's 1932 article, he attacked notions that Spanish-speaking children were inherently intellectually inferior to English-speaking American children as indicated by IQ scores (Sanchez, 1932). He was the first who brought into serious question the interpretation of heredity as the primary basis for observed differences in IQ scores. Dr. Sanchez strongly criticized the misuse and misapplication of psychological tests when measuring intelligence and of those who ignored bilingual and cultural factors. He argued that the worth of any test instrument lies in its proper interpretation and its ability to meet the educational needs of students (Sanchez, 1934). Dr. Sanchez was among the first to actively promote bilingual and bicultural educational programs, which later provided the foundation for present-day Headstart programs.

Almost 100 years later, the concerns raised by Dr. George Sanchez persist even though improvements have been made. The field of psychological testing continues to advance and testing instruments continue to improve, with revision after revision including most representative standardized samples in their work. Many clinicians have made modifications in the administration and interpretation of standardized psychological measures as mentioned previously. The value of modifying or altering a test may provide important qualitative information and enhance clinical utility such as through direct observations of testing behavior, assessment of learning propensity, evaluation of developmental capabilities, and error analysis (Ortiz and Menlo, 2015). Ortiz and Menlo (2015) highlight the value and richness of this information for intervention planning and remediation purposes. However, following standardized methods and instruction is crucial at first. If validity concerns are present, then obtaining qualitative information may be beneficial, and any changes to standardized procedures should be noted in the assessment report.

Nonverbal Intellectual Testing

Another alternative that psychologists and other testing clinicians have resorted to when working with Spanish-speaking Latinx persons has entailed the use of nonverbal intellectual testing. This is a popular method of assessment because of the idea of eliminating the perceived language barrier, and thereby producing a reliable measure of cognitive functioning, is attractive to practitioners (Ortiz, Ochoa, & Dynda, 2012). However, concerns remain when relying on nonverbal measures for intelligence testing. Lohman, Krob, and Laki (2008) argue that nonverbal measures are poor predictors of academic achievement. Ortiz and Menlo (2015) also highlight that nonverbal tests are not culture-free simply because language has been excluded in the assessment. For example, many nonverbal measures of intelligence rely on objects, pictures, and visual stimuli that come from a specific culture. Thus, non-majority individuals may be at a disadvantage. Furthermore, nonverbal measures suffer from construct underrepresentation with regard to intelligence because they only assess a narrow range of cognitive abilities and processes compared to batteries that include verbal and nonverbal subtests. This underrepresentation will then create an obstacle when evaluating disorders in which deficiencies in specific cognitive domains and/or processes are necessary for diagnosis, such as specific learning disabilities. Therefore, it is important to closely examine the referral question at hand when determining if a nonverbal assessment is sufficient. Relying on nonverbal tests exclusively when working with a Latinx client is not a best practice.

Having a bilingual psychologist administer a native-language intellectual assessment seems to be the ideal scenario. However, Ortiz and Menlo (2015) point out that validity concerns may still persist because a scarcity of research exists regarding intellectual testing among Latinx persons with varying levels of Spanish and English proficiency. One concern is that most Spanish native assessments are normed outside the United States on Spanish-speaking populations who normally come from one country and speak, learn, and are educated in that same language. These populations are quite different from Latinx people in the United States, who are exposed to two cultures, at least two languages, and receive their education in English or in bilingual formats. Thus, English proficiency and acculturation are concerns in Spanish-language assessments. Ortiz and Menlo (2015) note that simply speaking the native language of the examinee does not suffice for equitable and fair evaluations of Latinx persons and, in fact, that the psychometric properties of assessments used and the examinee's language proficiency and acculturation affect test performance. Clinician knowledge in the interaction of language and education received and understanding how linguistic, cognitive, and educational development play a role in test performance is most critical. Additionally, integrating these factors within a theoretically guided and empirically supported framework is important (Geisinger & Carlton, 1998; Ortiz & Menlo, 2015). While gradual improvement in the training and expertise of individuals conducting these assessments has occurred over time, challenges continue to remain in regard to validity of measures, bias in English-to-Spanish adapted tests, tests not being updated or having small/nonrepresentative samples, tests not meeting full criteria for standards of assessments, and access to care for the Latinx population (Puente et al., 2015).

Some researchers have surveyed the popularity of certain cognitive measures used with Latinx clients. Renteria (2010) noted that most commonly used cognitive assessment include the Ravens Coloured Progressive Matrices (Raven, 2003); the Test of Nonverbal Intelligence, Third Edition; the Bateria Woodcock Muñoz; the Bateria Neuropsicologica en Espanol; and the NUEROPSI-Attention and Memory, and others. Puente et al. (2015) also reported results from a more recent survey conducted with the Hispanic Neuropsychological Society (HNS) highlighting the most used Spanish measures. The survey results noted the top 25 Spanish measures; the top 5 included the Trail Making Test (TMT), Beck Depression Inventory (BDI-II), Boston Naming Test (BNT), Test of Memory and Malingering (TOMM), and the Beck Anxiety Inventory (BAI). The Minnesota Multiphasic Personality Inventory (MMPI2), Escala de Inteligencia de Weschler para Adultos (EIWA-III), and the Bateria III Woodcock Munoz also made the top 10 list (Puente et al., 2015). Out of the 25 most common Spanish assessments identified, only the Bateria III, MMPI2, WISCV, and the EIWAIII met the

Standards for Educational and Psychological Testing criteria of (a) test availability in Spanish, (b) Latinx US norms, (c) non-US Latinx norms, and (d) availability of a Spanish test manual. Many other Spanish measures identified had one to three criteria from these standards but failed to meet all four. Puente and colleagues (2015) urge that, as presented in the *Standards*, it is critical to assess the reliability and validity of tests currently available, develop norms for respective groups, revise current English-to-Spanish translations, increase Spanish-language and cultural awareness training, and address the needs and challenges of testing Spanish speakers.

The Council of National Psychological Associations for the Advancement of Ethnic Minority Interests (CNPAAEMI), a multinational association bringing together various ethnic minority psychological associations worked, in 2016, on a timely monograph on testing and assessment with people and communities of color. The monograph touched on different cultures and highlighted culture-specific tools one may use when assessing Latinx clients and other groups, such as African American, Native American, and Asian Americans. For Latinx persons, the authors mentioned specific measures that are considered best practice given the reliability and validity with Latinx samples (CNPAAEMI, 2016). For example, the Neuropsychological Screening for Hispanics (NeSBHIS) is a fairly new measure created for and normed with Latinx people.

Cognitive Test Descriptions

Batería III Woodcock-Muñoz (Batería IV). The Bateria IV is a comprehensive assessment that evaluates individuals whose native language is Spanish. It facilitates exploration of strengths and weaknesses across cognitive, linguistic, and academic abilities and goes beyond CHC theory as conceived in the Bateria III. The Batería III was the Spanish adaptation of the Woodcock-Johnson III (WJ-III; Munoz-Sandoval et al., 2005). It was created by directly translating instructions of certain tests from the WJ-III while adapting others for use with Spanish speakers. This test was normed on 1,413 native Spanish-speaking individuals from inside and outside the United States, including Mexico, Central America, South America, and Spain. Like the WJ-III, the Batería III has both cognitive and achievement batteries and can be used with individuals between 2 and 90 years of age. The Batería Woodcock Munoz is based on a model of intellectual ability highlighting four groups of cognitive abilities including acquired knowledge, short-term memory, thinking abilities, and facilitators-inhibitors (Geisinger, 2015). The manual includes norms from the different countries of origin. Overall, the factor loadings of the Batería III indicate a good relationship with the internal factor structure of the WJ-III (Curiel et al., 2016). The Batería IV provides an efficient and psychometrically sound assessment of cognitive and academic skills with updated norms and content that reflect current Spanish linguistic culture. It is a useful battery used to assess cognitive functioning in Latinx groups who are not fully acculturated or not proficient in the English language.

Wechsler Adult Intelligence Scale-IV (WAIS-IV). The WAIS-IV is an adult measure of cognitive ability based on research in the area of cognitive neuroscience and the theories and work by Wechsler (WAIS-IV, 2008). This measure produces scores along four indices: the verbal comprehension index, the perceptual reasoning index, the working memory index, and the processing speed index. Each index comprises a number of different subtests covering major categories of cognitive functioning. The WAIS-IV was standardized on an English-speaking population that was stratified to match US demographics. Extremely limited research has explored the impact of acculturation on WAIS-IV performance and the validity of this cognitive measure with Latinx individuals. Weiss et al. (2010) published preliminary data that seem to indicate that WAIS-IV scores are less impacted by ethnicity compared to the WAIS-III (Wechsler, 1997) and are instead more affected by education. However, it is very important to be cautious when interpreting the WAIS-IV with Latinx clients, as those not fully acculturated may have discrepancies in scores. That is why assessing acculturation in the beginning phase of the assessment is important to adequately decide what cognitive instrument to use.

Escala de Intelligencia de Wechsler para Adultos (EIWA). The original EIWA was standardized on 1,127 native Puerto Ricans between 16 and 64 years of age. The EIWA's subtests are similar to the WAIS scales, and the EIWA was found to be reliable, with coefficient alphas ranging from .65 to .96 for subtests and .95 to .98 for composite scores. The EIWA is a Spanish version of the original WAIS; research has demonstrated equivalent factor structure and adequate reliability and psychometric properties (Maldonado & Geisinger, 2005). Still, research by Lopez and Romero (1988) and Melendez (1994) did identify an overestimation of IQ scores for Latinx persons. Formal and informal evidence has indicated that there is an inflation of IQs for Latinx individuals when compared to scores from English-language measures or when developed cognitive abilities were estimated from known levels of functioning (Geisinger, 2015). To address some of the concerns from the original EIWA and EIWA-II, the EIWA III revision's norms were based on 2,450 individuals from across the United States, ranging from 16 to 89 years of age with equal numbers of men and women and racial group balances. Adequate reliability and validity coefficients were reported (Geisinger, 2005). Given that the standardization of the EIWA is with the Puerto Rican population, one must be cautious when administering the EIWA to other Latinx groups. The items in Verbal Comprehension, for example, are specific to the Puerto Rican culture, and a client from another Latinx group would struggle in the Vocabulary and Information subtests, thus compromising estimation of their true cognitive functioning.

Wechsler Intelligence Scale for Children Fifth Edition (WISC-V Spain). A revised and adapted version of the US WISC-V (Wechsler, 2014) was recently published in Spain, the Escala de inteligencia de Wechsler para niños–V (WISC-V Spain; Wechsler, 2015). Fenollar-Cortés and Watkins (2019) examined the construct validity of this Spanish version WISC-V employing confirmatory factor analysis (CFA). For all 15 subtests, the higher-order model proposed by Wechsler

(2015) contained five group factors but lacked discriminant validity. This study found that a traditional Wechsler four-factor structure was more appropriate when best-practice CFA methods were applied. The authors concluded that the cumulative weight of reliability and validity evidence supported the general factor level but that extreme caution should be used when using group factor scores to make decisions about individual children. Previous versions like the WISC-R were adapted into three Spanish versions for Puerto Rico, Spain, and Mexico, and the WISC-III was later adapted for Argentina (Geisinger, 2015). The WISC-IV reported sound psychometric properties, and most recent WISC-V-Spain, published in 2015, also noted appropriate psychometric properties (Fenollar-Cortes & Watkins, 2019). The WISC has been adapted because of different semantic variations in target populations. Different norms exist for the various WISC Spanish versions, such as for Spain, Mexico, and Puerto Rico (Sanchez-Escobedo, Hollingworth, & Fina, 2011). It is important to select the appropriate edition of both the test and the norms for the target population to ensure that scores are interpreted in their cultural context.

Mexican WAIS-III. Limited psychometric research exists for the Mexican Wechsler Adult Intelligence Scale-Third Edition (Mexican WAIS-III). The Mexican WAIS-III was normed on 970 Mexican individuals, and both US and Mexican norms are available for clinicians to interpret. Concerns regarding representative sample, subtest reliability, lack of psychometric score normalization, and direct translation of WAIS-III content have been voiced (Suen & Greenspan, 2009). Therefore, clinicians should practice caution when interpreting the WAIS-III with Latinx groups specifically from Mexican descent.

Neuropsychological Screening Battery for Hispanics. Another instrument that was normed for the Latinx population was the Neuropsychological Screening Battery for Hispanics (NeSBHIS). The NeSBHIS was created by Ponton et al. (2000) to measure language memory, attention, motor, and visual spatial functioning in Latinx Spanish speakers aged 16 to 75. This measure was normed on representative numbers of Latinx persons, making it a unique assessment with rich normative data. This assessment is one measure developed for and normed with the Latinx population representing robust construct validity (Ponton et al., 2000).

Many of the cognitive measures discussed in this section were developed for Spanish-speaking populations and are administered in Spanish. As discussed previously, when a Spanish-speaking client needs to be assessed cognitively, a best practice is for the client to be assessed by a Spanish-speaking examiner using a validated Spanish edition of a cognitive test. When the examiner is not Spanish-speaking, an interpreter is warranted. Clinicians need to use caution when using interpreters, and they must be aware of the ethical guidelines for the use of interpreters and assure that the general guidelines for selection, training, and use of interpreters are followed. For example, when examiners rely on untrained translators, the psychological assessment may become ineffective and may affect the validity of test scores. (Please see "Working with Interpreters" in Chapter 6 for more information on guidelines for using interpreters in psychological assessment.)

PERSONALITY MEASURES

There has been a rise in attention to cultural competency in psychological assessment, but the quality and quantity of research does not match the current
need for information. Studies on culturally diverse groups are scarce for many
popular psychological measures, ranging from the well-researched Personality
Assessment Inventory (PAI; Morey, 20114), to projective techniques like the
Thematic Apperception Test (Miller & Loveler, 2020). In this section, we discuss
projective tests and non-projective personality assessment instruments.

Projective Tests

Some psychologists refrain from using projective measures due to concerns about
validity and reliability. However, some find significant clinical utility with the
data that collected during the assessment. The Rorschach Inkblot test is one projective measure used to identify personality disorders and assess for emotional
functioning. The Rorschach Inkblot projective test consists of 10 inkblots printed
on cards; examinees are asked what they see by the clinician. The Exner scoring
system is a comprehensive approach to coding the quality of each response that
pays attention to form, movement, color, shading, pairs, and reflections. Some
psychologists use it for ruling out psychotic disorders. Research studies on the
Rorschach Inkblot test indicate significant concerns with culturally diverse
groups. Miller and Loveler (2020) noted that several studies indicate that scores
for community samples of Mexicans, Central Americans, and South Americans
on the Rorschach test often differ significantly from norms of the Exner system
for scoring this test, raising concern regarding whether the test can be used with
ethnically diverse groups in the United States (Wood et al., 2003). However, other
researchers have postulated that the Rorschach comprehensive system includes
inkblots that have universal meanings, such as extraversion-introversion system
constructs that include facets of activity, assertiveness, excitement-seeking,
warmth, and positive emotions (Dana, 1993). Cross-cultural research on the
Rorschach in Latin America and Europe noted shared common worldview and
cultural values (Meyers, Erdberg, & Shaffer, 2015). Other studies in many countries strongly suggests that the Rorschach test overpathologizes multicultural
populations living in the United States (Dana, 2013). It is clear that multicultural
research on the Rorschach is critical, and continued research focusing on diverse
community and clinical groups is timely and essential.

The Thematic Apperception Test (TAT) is another projective personality
measure that is commonly used with culturally diverse groups. TAT research has
supported its use with monocultural and multicultural populations. Objective
TAT scores were originally developed in the United States for 12 cards used with
national normative data (Ávila-Espada, 2000). The TAT also has a Spanish translation using a psychocultural scoring system, which includes an anthropological
scoring guide highlighting human motivation and personality, and local norms

(Ephraim, Sochting, & Marcia, 1997). Jenkins (2008) developed a handbook of TAT scores and scoring systems for perceptual–cognitive, psychodynamic, and socioemotional variables to encourage future TAT research and eventual application as a more useful instrument for personality assessment. Jenkins's (2008) handbook of monocultural objective scores and multicultural and cross-cultural groups also included children and TAT-derived instruments like the Tell-Me-a-Story Test (TEMAS), thus offering a culturally sensitive scoring guide. The TAT's combined research and practice guidelines enhance reliability and use with culturally diverse groups (Dana, 2003). Furthermore, additional TAT multicultural application studies conducted by Avila-Espada (2000) and Ephraim (2000) have furthered TAT's use with culturally diverse groups. For example, Avila-Espada's (2000) research on the TAT using US and Spanish norms noted low language interference in interpretation for the Latinx populations, and Ephraim (2000) emphasized an etic-emic psychocultural research and practice model with 10 basic Murray cards with Latinx groups. Despite some promising research on the TAT cards used with culturally diverse populations like Latinx people, there is still a need for adoption of new culture-specific sets of cards for Latinx, African American, Asian American, and Anglo American populations (Dana, 1999).

TEMAS. The TEMAS ("*Temas*" means "themes" in Spanish) is a multicultural thematic apperception test developed for minority and non-minority youth aged 5 to 18 years. The TEMAS is an effective tool for Latinx youth and children of color (Malgady, Costantino, & Rogler, 1984). It includes brightly colored pictures of Latinx and African American characters in different situations in urban settings. The TEMAS is a popular projective measure because it was developed and normed for the Latinx population. It measures some dynamics of personality and cognitive and affective functioning in children and adolescents (CNPAAEMI, 2016). CNPAAEMI (2016) noted that the TEMAS is a culturally relevant assessment that was created for Latinx persons and not adapted and that it should be a model for future assessment development. Despite its acceptable psychometrics, it is still underutilized (Dana, 2015). Barriers to utilization of the TEMAS may include lack of clinician knowledge of the TEMAS and inadequate clinical training practices.

Minnesota Multiphasic Personality Inventory-2 (MMPI-2). The MMPI-2 has some positive indicators for use with Latinx persons and other people of color. The MMPI-2 was originally developed in the 1930s at the University of Minnesota to help identify psychopathology including personal, social, and behavioral problems in psychiatric populations. As in many assessments, the initial version mostly included White, middle-class groups in the standardization group. Recent research, however, posits that the revised MMPI-2 is a suitable measure for Black and Latinx populations in the United States because the distribution of scores in these groups is similar to the distribution of scores for Whites. Wood and colleagues (2003) highlight that the revisions of the original MMPI provide a model for improving older tests that are not suitable for use with minority populations. Of course, the MMPI-2 has improved in its standardization and, in particular, in the inclusion of ethnic minority groups. Revisions of the MMPI-2 for noted deficiencies include items, norms, flawed psychometric properties, and construct changes (Ranson, Nichols, Rouse, & Harrington, 2009).

The MMPI-2 has been translated into Spanish in several versions, and some have demonstrated strong psychometric validity (Boscan et al, 2000; Butcher et al., 2007). Velasquez et al. (2000) put forth important cautionary guidelines when using the MMPI-2 with culturally diverse groups. For instance, they recommend assuring a standardized procedure in its administration and being cautious when using computerized interpretive reports. Additionally, the clinician must be careful when interpreting clinical and validity scales, and considering the role of cultural values and acculturation, including acculturative stress, is imperative. It is essentially the responsibility of the psychologist to individualize interpretations to cultural factors in order to avoid overpathologizing. When interpreting personality measures like the MMPI-2, it is imperative to understand the role that cultural values may play in perhaps influencing the elevation of clinical and validity scales. For example, in the United States, Latinx persons tend to score higher than the normative sample on the F and L scales (Whitworth & McBlaine, 1993). The normative sample of the MMPI-2 included 2,600 individuals (1,138 males and 1,462 females) age 18 and older. Multiple racial and ethnic groups were included in the normative sample, but no separate cultural norms are available. The F scale is intended to detect unusual or atypical ways of answering test items, whereas the L scale detects individuals answering untruthfully.

The MMPI-2 is the most widely used and frequently researched self-report personality inventory, and it has demonstrated its clinical utility and applicability with Spanish-speaking Latinx populations in the United States as well as in several Spanish-speaking countries (Garrido & Cabiya, 2013). It should be noted that the existing norms for the MMPI-2 include only a small and unrepresentative sample of Spanish speakers ($n = 73$) limited to one region of the United States. Despite this limitation, research studies comparing MMPI-2 profiles of Latinx to non-Latinx White examinees have found that, although differences in profiles exist, these are small (e.g., Hall et al., 1999; Whitworth & McBlaine, 1993). Moreover, the MMPI-2 has been translated into different Spanish versions for regional use, including Spain (Castilian), Mexico, Central America, and Spanish for the United States. Current literature supports the reliability and validity of the English version of the MMPI-2 (Ben-Porath & Tellegen, 2008), but few studies have examined the reliability and validity of the Spanish versions.

One of the first research studies examining different Spanish versions of the MMPI-2 with Latinx samples outside the United States compared Puerto Rican, Mexican, and US Latinx college students (Cabiya et al., 2000). The Puerto Rican sample consisted of 271 students (149 males and 122 females) who were administered the Chilean version of the MMPI-2 (Rissetti et al., 1996), the Mexican sample included 2,174 students (929 males and 1,245 females) who were administered the Mexican version of the MMPI-2 (Lucio & Reyes, 1994; Lucio et al., 1994), and the US sample consisted of 1,312 college students (515 males and 797 females) who were administered the US-Spanish translation (Garcia-Peltoniemi & Azan-Chaviano, 1993). No significant differences between the two

Latinx samples outside the United States were found across the validity and clinical scales. Similarly, no differences were found between the sample of Puerto Rican college students and the US Latinx sample except with regard to the Masculinity/ Femininity (Mf) scale. In light of the absence of significant differences among the three groups, the authors endorsed the appropriateness of such translations and adaptions of the MMPI-2 for their use in Latin America.

Overall, Handel and Ben-Porath (2000) endorse the general equivalence of existing translated versions of the MMPI-2 to the original measure. Nevertheless, they maintain that the development of local norms should be considered, particularly given the substantial variability within cultures among Spanish-speakers. Accordingly, Lucio and colleagues (1999, 2001) developed language adaptations and corresponding norms for the MMPI-2 and its adolescent version, the MMPI-A, in Mexico. These researchers investigated the adequacy of existing MMPI-2 norms for the MMPI-2 translated version for Mexico. They concluded that although the local norms were similar to the US norms, local norms were more capable of accounting for cultural factors. For example, Mexican test-takers may frequently endorse items related to spirituality, elevating their scores in the Schizophrenia (Sc) and the Bizarre Mentation (BIZ) scales. The influence of cultural values should be taken into account in understanding this pattern of responses to avoid overpathologizing this population.

In summary, while there is a dearth of research examining the validity, reliability, equivalence, or bias of MMPI-2 translated or adapted versions for use with Latinx individuals, the extant evidence reveals few and relatively small differences between Latinx individuals and non-Latinx White individuals on MMPI-2 scales. Indeed, Butcher and coauthors (2007) have published work validating the appropriateness of the use of adaptations of the MMPI-2 and the MMPI-A with Latinx clients.

The MMPI-2-RF is the most recent version of the MMPI-2. This restructured form contains 338 items, 9 validity scales, 51 empirically validated scales, and 8 restructured clinical (RC) scales (Dana, 2013). It is important to note there are three Spanish versions of the MMPI-2-RF: Spanish for Mexico and Central America; Spanish for Spain, South America, and Central America (Castilian); and Spanish for the United States. We focus on the development of the US Spanish version; however, each Spanish version for regional use underwent similar procedures for translation and standardization. Each Spanish translation is listed on the University of Minnesota Press website (https://www.upress.umn.edu/test-division/translations-permissions/available-translations) and is available for purchase through separate retailers (University of Minnesota Press, 2011–2020).

US Spanish MMPI-2-RF. The MMPI-Hispana paved the way for the US Spanish MMPI-2-RF. The US Spanish version of the MMPI-2-RF was created using the Spanish items of the MMPI-Hispana, in a similar procedure as used when creating the MMPI-2-RF scales from the MMPI-2. In other words, the current US Spanish MMPI-2-RF was created from an extracted item pool of the MMPI-Hispana. One of the major questions about the original MMPI and MMPI-Hispana was if the measures feature inherent ethnic bias and are applicable for cross-cultural use. Research on the MMPI-Hispana is mixed, with some evidence of overpathologizing Latinx respondents and other work suggesting comparability (Butcher et al., 2007; Greene, 1987; Velasquez et al., 1997; Velasquez, 2000). Specifically, a review conducted by Green (1987) found an overall tendency on the MMPI-2/MMPI-Hispana for Latinx individuals to score higher than White respondents on L (e.g., untruthful responses) and F (e.g., atypical responses) scales.

There is limited research on the MMPI-2-RF Spanish version. One of the earliest studies on the US Spanish MMPI-2-RF compared MMPI-Hispana scales to extracted MMPI-2-RF scales in Latinx respondents with depression (Khouri, 2010). The primary goal of the study was to determine if depression difficulties manifested in a comparable manner across the two forms. Results indicated more scale elevations on the MMPI-2-RF scales, specifically Infrequent Responses, Infrequent Somatic Responses, Symptom Validity, Malaise, Neurological Complaints, Cognitive Complaints, and Anxiety as compared with the MMPI-2-RF. Authors determined that this difference across the two versions suggested that use of the MMPI-2-RF with Latinx respondents was "premature"; however, the difference could also be interpreted as improved sensitivity to pathological symptoms of depression within the MMPI-2-RF.

Kermott (2017) examined comparability of the English MMPI-2-RF with the US Spanish MMPI-2-RF and a smaller sample of the Castilian version. Participants ($N = 63$) were bilingual adults living in southern California. Subjects were administered both the English and US Spanish MMPI-2-RFs, with 22 respondents also administered the Castilian version in a single session. Mean results on all scales were then compared using analysis of variance (ANOVA) tests. Analyses comparing the scale means of the US Spanish and English versions failed to indicate significant group differences, which the researcher suggested implies comparability of the two versions. Because of the limited amount of research on the MMPI-2-RF, it is difficult to draw conclusions regarding how the measure functions within Latinx populations; however, early evidence is promising.

Spanish MMPI-3. Special considerations by the MMPI-3 authors was taken to ensure that this measure will be culturally sensitive and appropriate. Similar to the upcoming MMPI-3, the US Spanish MMPI-3 will feature an updated norming sample. For the first time, the MMPI-3 team gathered data not only on ethnically diverse, but also linguistically diverse individuals to ensure appropriate representation of Latinx persons in the standardization sample (Ben-Porath & Tellegen, 2008). The sample will include 45 bilingual individuals for comparison in addition to 664 Spanish-speaking monolinguals. Additionally, the upcoming MMPI-3 will reword some of the previously noted problematic items. Existing items of concern, in addition to the new items, were translated by Dr. Antonio Puente at University of North Carolina-Wilmington (Ben-Porath & Tellegen, 2008).

The MMPI-3 will include a specific manual for the US Spanish version for the first time (Hall, Menton, & Ben-Porath, 2022). This manual features a thorough history of the development of the US Spanish MMPI-3, as well as norming information and instructions on how to accurately use the measure, including its administration, scoring, and interpretation. It is important to note that some of the data collected for the proposed study are included in the manual's reliability and validity calculations in addition to data collected through various projects. Currently, the sample in the manual includes 1,098 individuals and will most likely be updated in the forthcoming publication. Taken together, it is clear that the MMPI-3 is proactively addressing concerns of ethnic or linguistic bias within the previous editions and may be a promising instrument for the assessment of Latinx persons.

Personality Assessment Inventory (PAI). The PAI is a self-administered objective test of personality and psychopathology published by Morey in 1991, and extensively used in clinical settings. This test consists of four sets of scales: 4 validity scales, 11 clinical scales covering major categories of pathology corresponding to DSM-IV (APA, 1994), 5 treatment consideration scales, and 2 interpersonal scales. In addition to the original instrument, there are Spanish and adolescent (PAI-A) versions available. The PAI has demonstrated good psychometric properties (i.e., convergent and discriminant validity, internal consistency, and test-retest reliability) and content validity (Morey, 1991); however, only a few studies have explored the psychometric properties of the PAI with Latinx populations.

An early study conducted by Rogers et al. (1995) examined equivalence between the Spanish and English versions of the PAI as well as the test-retest reliability of the Spanish version with a predominantly Mexican American sample ($N = 69$). Their results revealed moderate to good correlations on the clinical scales ($Mr = .71$) between the English and Spanish versions, good stability (test-retest) for the clinical scales in Spanish version ($Mr = .78$), and modest to good internal consistency for Latinx respondents on both the Spanish and English versions. In contrast, the authors found substantial variations in the equivalence and consistency of scores regarding the validity, treatment, and interpersonal scales. In view of these results, the researchers caution that interpretation of the results of these scales may not be valid.

Fernandez and colleagues (2008) investigated the ability of the PAI validity scales to identify under- and overreporting of pathology on both the English and Spanish versions of the PAI. The researchers administered both language versions of the PAI to a sample of 72 bilingual participants under instructions to respond honestly, to overreport psychopathology, or to underreport psychopathology. The English and Spanish versions' validity scales performed similarly, and scores from the Negative Impression Management and the Positive Impression Management scales showed the highest levels of correspondence and accuracy for the identification of feigning across language versions. On the other hand, the other scales demonstrated either significant mean differences or low correlations across the English and Spanish versions. Furthermore, a trend was observed for underreporting scales to be elevated when participants responded honestly to the Spanish version of the PAI. The authors summarized that their findings support the appropriateness of the Spanish translation of the PAI.

More recently, a study conducted by Estrada and Smith (2019) compared the scores of Latinx and non-Latinx White college students on selected scales of the PAI. Findings from this study revealed that Latinx participants obtained significantly higher scores compared to the non-Latinx White participants on the INF (Infrequency), ARD (Anxiety Related Disorders), PAR (Paranoia), SCZ (Schizophrenia), NON (Non-Support), and STR (Stress) scales. Latinx participants also obtained scores indicative of greater psychological distress and psychopathology (MCE) than their counterparts. Furthermore, non-Latinx White participants obtained higher WRM (Interpersonal Warmth) scores, contrary to the initial hypothesis of the researchers. Given their findings, the authors call on psychologists to exercise caution when interpreting PAI results of Latinx clients in clinical settings.

TRAUMA ASSESSMENTS

Trauma assessment among Latinx populations living in the United States is a critical need, and all mental health practitioners should be aware of the particularly high risk for trauma exposure and persistent posttraumatic symptoms present among Latinx immigrants. Indeed, 60% of Latinx immigrant youth experience clinically significant posttraumatic stress symptoms (Venta & Mercado, 2019), in contrast to less than 15% in non-immigrant groups (Foa et al., 2001), with the mean level of posttraumatic stress symptoms 161% higher in Latinx immigrant children and 204% higher in Latinx immigrant adolescents than in non-immigrants (Venta & Mercado, 2018). Not surprisingly, these levels of posttraumatic symptomology mirror very high levels of trauma exposure in teens: seeing someone in the community get slapped, punched, or beaten up (64%); experiencing a serious accident or injury (56%); experiencing a natural disaster (51%); witnessing violence perpetrated against a family member (45%); and, in children (by parent-report), seeing someone in the community get slapped, punched, or beaten up (39%); experiencing a natural disaster (27%); witnessing violence perpetrated against a family member (25%); and experiencing a serious accident or injury (25%; Venta & Mercado, 2018).

Pre-migration, immigrants face risk factors including peer delinquency; peer rejection; poor parental management; lack of social support; community disorganization (Borum, Bartel, & Forth, 2006); a history of poverty; exposure to violence, political chaos, and discrimination (Kennedy & Ceballo, 2014; Stinchcomb & Hershberg, 2014); having been persecuted or fearing persecution; experiencing or witnessing violence, murders, and social chaos (Hodes, 2000); and having been sexually abused, physically abused, or tortured (Edwards & Beiser, 1994). Indeed, Central American countries, a large source of Latinx migration to the United States in recent years, have high rates of violence, poverty, drug trafficking, and organized crime, all contributing to migration outflow from these regions (Rosenblum & Ball, 2016). Additionally, migration-related risk factors include robbery, physical, sexual assaults at the hands of *coyotes* (i.e., immigrant smugglers), pursuit by government officials, food deprivation, dehydration, and witnessing murder, rape, and assault (Suárez-Orozco, 2001). Some of the little empirical data available in recently immigrated youth samples indicate that 24–29.8% of children report experiencing traumatic events during migration to the United States (Perreira & Ornelas, 2013; Vasquez-Guzman et al., 2020) and that the majority of in-transit traumatic events (82.1%) are not captured by standard trauma assessment, indicating significant limitations in existing instruments (Vasquez-Guzman et al., 2020). Certainly, post-migration stressors may also increase risk for trauma exposure and posttraumatic symptoms among immigrant Latinx persons as well as second-generation Latinx persons living in the United States. These stressors can include, but are not limited to, continued victimization, financial adversities, difficulties in planning relocation (Saldana, 1992; Yearwood, Crawford, Kelly, & Moreno, 2007), and stress from leaving behind family and social support (Patel, Clarke, Eltareb, Macciomei, & Wickham, 2016). Additionally, coping with the double stigma of being outsiders and "illegal aliens" poses an additional stressor (Alba & Nee, 2005; Ferraro, 2013).

Trauma Assessment in Children

Among measures assessing exposure to potentially traumatic events, Part I of the University of California Los Angeles (UCLA) posttraumatic stress disorder (PTSD) Index Trauma Screen – Revision 1 (UCLA PTSD; Pynoos, Rodriguez, Steinberg, Studber, & Frederick, 1997) is among the most widely used. It includes child/adolescent and parent forms that utilize clear, parsimonious language to facilitate lifetime trauma exposure screening (Steinberg, Brymer, Decker, & Pynoos, 2004). The strong psychometric properties of this instrument in English have been widely reviewed elsewhere (e.g., Steinberg et al., 2004), and it has been translated to Spanish (Erolin, Wieling, & Parra, 2014) and also been utilized in immigrant samples (Allen, Cisneros, & Tellez, 2015; Beehler, Birman, & Campbell, 2012). Finally, Venta and Mercado (2019) examined the psychometric properties of the instrument in Spanish-speaking immigrant samples. While cross-cultural invariance studies are lacking, the UCLA PTSD is recommended as an instrument of trauma exposure in Latinx youth, with the caveat that it may suffer from the limitations for assessing in-transit trauma noted by Vasquez-Guzman et al. (2020) and limitations in the availability of measurement invariance data.

Regarding the assessment of posttraumatic stress symptoms, the Child PTSD Symptoms Scale (CPSS; Foa, Johnson, Feeny, & Treadwell, 2001) is a questionnaire-based measure that is widely used with both youth self-report and caregiver-report forms. Foa et al. (2001) initially evaluated the psychometric properties of this instrument using a sample of 75 children from California. Subsequent research translated the measure into Spanish (e.g., Kataoka et al., 2009) and reported on the use of the scale in Latinx (Gudiño & Rindlaub, 2014) and immigrant (Jaycox et al., 2002) youth. Gudiño and Rindlaub (2014) were the first to conduct a full psychometric evaluation of the CPSS in Spanish utilizing a sample of 161 Hispanic students in the United States. Their results indicated high rates of PTSD symptoms (*Mean* = 12.11, *SD* = 9.56) with 52.8% of subjects meeting the clinical cutoff of

11 suggested by the measure's original authors (i.e., Foa et al., 2001). Findings supported the internal consistency of the CPSS (*alpha* = .75), provided no evidence of a relation between CPSS and age, and indicated a significant gender effect, with females reporting higher symptoms. Convergent validity was supported via significant relations with violence exposure. Finally, results indicated that a three-factor structure best fit the CPSS data. While Gudiño and Rindlaub (2014) made large strides toward psychometric assessment of the Spanish CPSS, only 31 students in their sample completed the measure in Spanish. Kassam-Adams et al. (2013) added to this literature base by utilizing the CPSS in 225 Spanish-speaking youth with recent trauma exposure and reporting adequate internal consistency (*alpha* = .88) and concurrent validity. Several studies have also utilized the CPSS in immigrant samples. Jaycox et al. (2002), for instance, reported on the CPSS utilizing a large sample (*N* = 1,004) of immigrant children, of whom about half were from Spanish-speaking countries in Central or South America. The CPSS was administered in Spanish to these children, although descriptive data were reported for the whole sample only. Overall, the total CPSS score was high (*M* = 9.56, *SD* = 8.14) with a significantly higher number of symptoms reported among girls. No psychometric data were reported. In a sample of 229 young immigrants from Mexico and Central America, Kataoka et al. (2003) administered the child version of the CPSS as part of an intervention program and demonstrated adequate internal consistency (*alpha* = .89). Results indicated that 90% of children exceeded the clinical cutoff (using score of 11) for PTSD. Findings from Venta and Mercado (2019) from immigrant Latinx child and adolescent samples likewise noted very high symptom levels and adequate psychometric properties for this instrument, although some items appeared problematic and the authors called for future research, including cross-cultural invariance studies. Recently, psychometric data on the caregiver version of the CPSS, when used with Latinx caregivers, have been published, and this version shows promise (Marshall & Venta, 2021).

Trauma Assessment in Adults

The Trauma History Questionnaire (Heilemann et al., 2005), a 24-item checklist that asks adults whether they have experienced 24 possibly traumatic events, is a commonly utilized assessment of trauma exposure in English. Participants answer "yes" or "no" and, if they endorse the exposure, the questionnaire prompts for how many times those specific events occurred in their lifetime and how old they were at exposure. The Trauma History Questionnaire's psychometric properties have been well-documented, and the instrument has been translated into Spanish (Hooper et al., 2011). While it has been used with Latinx persons, including in a recent study of Spanish-speakers (Mercado, Venta, Henderson, & Pimentel, 2019) and in studies of Latinx English-speakers, its cross-cultural validity has not been evaluated to our knowledge.

Regarding assessment of posttraumatic stress symptoms in adults, the Harvard Trauma Questionnaire (Mollica et al., 1992) has likely received the greatest psychometric support across cultural groups, including Latinx populations. In addition to a large literature base supporting its use among English-speaking, US-born individuals, the Harvard Trauma Questionnaire is available in Spanish, and empirical evaluation by Rasmussen, Verkuilen, Ho, and Fan (2015) indicated that response patterns did not differ according to language of assessment. The authors also examined cross-cultural measurement invariance and did not report concerns regarding their small Latin American subgroup (Rasmussen et al., 2015).

Another commonly used instrument for the assessment of posttraumatic symptoms in adults is the 22-item Impact of Events Scale (Báguena et al., 2001). The 22 items identify symptoms of posttraumatic stress via a Likert-type scale ranging from 1 (never) to 5 (always), and the instrument has been published in Spanish, with reliability estimates of the total scale ranging from 0.91 to 0.95 (Báguena et al., 2001). Mercado, Venta, Henderson, and Pimentel (2019) reported on this instrument in a sample of Spanish-speaking, recently immigrated adults from Latin America. Internal consistency in that sample was excellent ($\alpha = 0.91$), and the mean level of symptoms reported was high (59.72, $SD = 22.76$). Furthermore, factor analytic research with Latinx respondents is promising. Still, to our knowledge, no measurement invariance work has examined language of administration or cultural group of respondents for this instrument.

YOUTH PSYCHOPATHOLOGY MEASURES

There are a number of considerations when selecting youth psychopathology measures for use with Latinx youth. First, the existence of published basic psychometric properties relating to reliability and validity is critical for any psychological instrument. When working with Latinx persons, this point is further complicated by the sample in question—Latinx persons in the US in general, Spanish-speakers, Latinx English-speakers, Latinx persons who speak a language other than Spanish, or Spanish speakers/Hispanics living outside the United States. A second consideration relates to the more in-depth, cross-cultural psychometric properties discussed in Chapter 4. In this section we review commonly used youth psychopathology measures and consider these two matters. While the current section is focused on broad-band youth psychopathology measures and some of the most commonly used narrow-band scales, clinicians with a particular interest in specific narrow-band scales not described here are referred to Pina and colleagues' (2013) comprehensive review of existing literature in their chapter "Toward Evidence-Based Clinical Assessment of Ethnic Minority Youth."

Achenbach System of Empirically Based Assessment. The Achenbach System of Empirically Based Assessment (ASEBA; Achenbach & Rescorla, 2000), which includes the Youth Self-Report, the Child Behavior Checklist, and the Teacher Report Form, is a well-known and often-used broad-band assessment of children's internalizing and externalizing psychopathology. The various ASEBA forms cover infancy through the age of 18, and reliability and validity data were adequate both in the initial publication manual (Achenbach & Rescorla, 2001) and in a copious amount of research that has followed. Research on the English versions of the ASEBA instruments with Latinx youth is predictably more limited but generally demonstrates adequate psychometric properties on various ASEBA versions reaching back to 1983 (see Zamarripa & Lerma, 2013). Another body of research has examined the Spanish versions of the ASEBA instruments, though much of this literature uses non-US samples. Early research indicated some problems with the Spanish translations: namely, that items have different meanings in Spanish than in English (Casas et al., 1998), though research with the more recently translated versions has demonstrated equivalence between Spanish and English versions (Gross et al.,2006).

Behavior Assessment System for Children. The Behavior Assessment System for Children (BASC; Reynolds & Kamphaus, 2004) is a second widely used broad-band measure of internalizing and externalizing symptoms in children, with Teacher Rating Scales, Parent Rating Scales, and Self-Report of Personality. Like the ASEBA scales, there is a large body of published work on the reliability and validity of BASC scales, with more limited literature on its use with English-speaking Latinx persons and even less on the Spanish translations. Research on an earlier Spanish version was promising (McCloskey et al., 2003), but research is lacking with the more recent second and third editions of the BASC.

Narrow-Band Scales. A number of narrow-band scales have documented reliability and validity data in Latinx samples. For internalizing symptoms, the Center for Epidemiologic Studies Depression Scale (Eaton et al., 2004), the Children's Depression Inventory, the Fear Survey Schedule for Children – Revised, the Multidimensional Anxiety Scale for Children, the Revised Children's Manifest Anxiety Scale, the Reynolds Adolescent Depression Scale, and the Social Phobia and Anxiety Inventory for Children have documented reliability and validity studies with Latinx persons (Pina et al., 2013). For externalizing behavior problems, the field is narrower, with only the Eyeberg Child Behavior Inventory having published reliability and validity data (Pina et al., 2013).

Suicide Risk and Self-Injurious Behavior Assessment. Maqueo and Arenas-Landgrave (2013) provide an overview of extant instruments for assessing suicide and self-injurious behavior risk among Hispanic adolescents. The findings from their review are troubling, indicating that there is no single measure for which adequate psychometric research has been published with adolescents in both Spanish and English. The Columbia Suicide Screen (Shaffer et al., 2004) is not recommended for use with Latinx adolescents; the Suicidal Ideation Questionnaire (Reynolds, 1987, 1991) is recommended for use with English-speaking Latinx persons only, in the absence of a Spanish translation; and the Beck Suicidal Ideation Scale (Beck & Steer, 1991), while available in Spanish, poses some validity concerns. Maqueo and Arenas-Landgrave's (2013) review of assessments of self-injurious behavior also reveals a concerning lack of available measures. The Self-Harm Behavior Questionnaire (Gutierrez et al. 2001) is recommended for use with English-speaking Latinx adolescents only, in the absence of a translation; and the Suicide Risk Inventory for Adolescents (also called the Inventario de Riesgo Suicida para Adolescentes; Hernandez & Lucio, 2006) is their recommended measure, with published data available in both Spanish and English.

CONCLUSION

Latinx groups in the United States have and continue to experience mental health disparities (Cardemil, 2010). In particular, psychological assessment with Latinx clients has been subjected to biases due to the use of psychological instruments not appropriate for this population. Biased psychological testing and assessment can be of great consequence, resulting in misdiagnosis which can lead to inappropriate services and treatment. For these reasons, the ethical and competent psychological assessment of Latinx individuals using appropriate tools is imperative. Accordingly, psychologists and clinicians who are trained in psychological testing should strive to use only psychological measures which have been established through research as valid for use with these population and carefully note when the state of the science prohibits this, interpreting their results with caution. In the same way, psychologists as a group should endeavor to adapt and develop assessment instruments with psychometric properties that enable appropriate and fair evaluation, diagnosis, and treatment planning of Latinx clients, particularly those whose English proficiency and acculturation levels differ from the mainstream population in the United States. Table 5.1 provides a summary of the personality, cognitive, and youth measures discussed in this chapter.

The works summarized in this chapter represent efforts by the psychology community toward such goal. Such efforts consist of research examining the equivalence and potential bias of available instruments when used with Latinx groups as well as translations and adaptations of existing measures. These research projects and innovations are largely being advanced by Latinx psychologists and their collaborators who draw from their expertise and personal knowledge of Latinx cultures with the goal of enhancing the amount and quality of resources available for psychological assessment with these groups. Nevertheless, it is clear that much work is still needed. Psychologists and other mental health clinicians and researchers should continue working to develop appropriate psychological instruments that are thoroughly adapted and normed for Latinx populations in order to ensure competent psychological assessment of these groups in the United States.

Table 5.1 SUMMARY OF ASSESSMENTS FOR SPANISH-SPEAKERS AND LATINX/MINORITY GROUPS

Assessment	Summary	Status/Recommendations
Cognitive		
Wechsler Adult Intelligence Scale-IV (WAIS-IV)	Cognitive assessment for adults It includes verbal comprehension, perceptual reasoning, working memory, and the processing speed subscales	Demonstrates adequate psychometric performance, but it was mostly standardized on Puerto Rican samples. Its Verbal Comprehension index is specific to Puerto Rican culture; caution is advised when administered to other Latinx groups.
Escala de Inteligencia de Weschler para Adultos (EIWA-III)	Cognitive assessment for adults with similar subtest to WAIS-IV	Demonstrates excellent internal validity and overall psychometric performance but overestimates IQ scores for Latinx persons.
Bateria III Woodcock Munoz: Prueba de Aprovechamiento	Assesses cognitive, linguistic, and academic abilities for ages 2–90; highlights cognitive abilities including acquired knowledge, short-term memory, thinking abilities, and facilitator-inhibitors	The assessment was validated on Spanish-speakers outside of the US and is normed by nationality.
Wechsler Intelligence Scale for Children Fifth Edition (WISC-V Spain) | the Escala de inteligencia de Wechsler para niños–V (WISC-V Spain)		Reports appropriate psychometric performance; clinicians must select correct norm and test contingent on Spain, Mexico, and Puerto Rico normed versions. Limitations must be considered when assessing other Latinx groups.
Mexican WAIS-III.	An adaptation of the WAIS-III, normed on 970 Mexican adults; the direct translation from the WAIS-III has been voided	High concerns about subset reliability and lack of psychometric score normalization. Caution is advised when administering this adaptation.
Neuropsychological Screening Battery for Hispanics (NeSBHIS)	The assessments measure language memory, attention, motor, and visual spatial function for clients aged 16–75	Validated on representative samples of Latinx groups and yielded robust construct validity. A trained Spanish interpreter is warranted for non-Spanish speakers.

Projective

Rorschach Inkblot test	A projective test used to identify personality disorders and emotional function and can be used to rule out psychotic disorders	High concerns with culturally diverse groups. Spanish-speakers' results differ significantly compared to those from the US.
Thematic Apperception Test	A projective personality measure consisting of 12 cards with normative scoring systems	Commonly used in diverse groups from mono- and multicultural backgrounds. A Spanish version is available with a corresponding scoring system and various local norms. More research is warranted to identify the assessment to specific minority groups.
Tell Me a Story (TEMAS)	A multicultural thematic apperception test for minority and non-minority minors aged 5–18; includes colored pictures of Latinx and African American characters as part of the materials; it measures dynamics of personality and cognitive and affection function	Has acceptable psychometrics but remains underutilized. TEMAS requires clinical training practices.

Personality and Psychopathology

MMPI-2	Measures psychopathology, personal, social and behavioral problems; Latinx persons living in the US score higher in the L and F scales; available norms include Spain, Mexico, Central America, and US Spanish	May be used with Black and Latinx persons given its ongoing standardization in minority samples. Spanish version demonstrates strong psychometric validity. Contextualizing acculturative stress, cultural values, standardized procedure, and computerized interpretive reports are critical when administering with minorities. Limited research has validated the psychometric performance of the various Spanish versions of the MMPI-2.

(*continued*)

Table 5.1 Continued

Assessment	Summary	Status/Recommendations
US Spanish MMPI-2-RF	The assessment was created from the MMPI-Hispana version	Virtually no psychometric research on this version on Latinx populations. Emerging research reveals positive results, but caution is warranted for clinicians given the limited research available.
Spanish MMP-3	The upcoming version of the MMPI will be updated and normed on a representative Latinx sample; it will reword previously identified problematic items	The MMPI-3 will include an US Spanish manual for the first time. It has addressed the major concerns of ethnic and linguistic bias in previous editions.
Personality Assessment Inventory	An objective test of personality and psychopathology with 11 clinical scales in accordance with the DSM-IV	Demonstrates good psychometric performance, but limited studies have verified such performance in Latinx samples. Latinx persons may score higher in INF, ARD, PAR, SCZ, NON, and STR scales compared to White samples; these warrant high caution when administering it to Latinx clients.
Trauma		Y
UCLA PTSD Index Trauma Screen - Revision 1	A child/adolescent and parent form that screens for trauma exposure	Has strong psychometrics properties in English. The Spanish version has psychometric limitation; it is highly recommended for Latinx youth, but special limitations apply for in-transit trauma screening.
Child PTSD Symptoms Scale	A caregiver and self-report form scale for PTSD symptoms, highly common in clinical settings	Revealed adequate internal consistency for US Hispanic children, but less research is available for other Latinx children from Central or South America. Caution is warranted as some items may be problematic, and because of lack of extant psychometric research on various Latinx children's samples.

Measure	Description	Notes
Trauma History Questionnaire	A 24-item checklist that screens for lifetime prevalence of traumatic events	Used in research settings but no research has identified its psychometric function with Latinx samples.
Harvard Trauma Questionnaire	A posttraumatic stress symptom screener for adults available for US-born English speakers and Spanish	Has the best psychometric performance in culturally diverse groups, including Latinx groups. The scales appear to be valid for various cross-cultural samples in Latin America.
Impact of Events Scale – 22.	A 22-item scale that screens for posttraumatic stress symptoms; available in English and Spanish	The scale reveals excellent internal consistency in immigrant and non-immigrant Spanish-speaking groups. Nonetheless, limitations are to be considered for limitations with language administration and for culturally diverse Spanish-speaking subgroups.
Youth Psychopathology		
Achenbach System of Empirically Based Assessments	Includes the Youth Self-Report, the Child Behavior Checklist, and the Teacher Report Forms used to assess internalizing and externalizing psychopathology in minors up to the age of 18	Limited research on the English version on Latinx children, but assessments revealed adequate psychometric performance. The most recently updated version revealed equivalency between the English and Spanish versions.
Behavior Assessment System for Children	A widely used measure of internalizing and externalizing symptomatology with teacher, parent, and self-report scales of personality	Very limited research on BASC psychometric performance in its English and Spanish versions with Latinx persons. These limitations must be considered when using in clinical settings.
Narrow-Band (Internalizing symptoms)	Children's Depression Inventory, Fear Survey Schedule for Children -Revised, Multidimensional Anxiety Scale for Children, Revised Children's Manifest Anxiety Scale, Reynolds Adolescent Depression Scale, and the Social Phobia and Anxiety Inventory for Children are narrow-band scales with available data on Latinx children to screen for internalizing symptomatology	These narrow-band scales demonstrate good reliability and validity in Latinx children.

(continued)

Table 5.1 Continued

Assessment	Summary	Status/Recommendations
Suicide & Self-Harm		
Columbia Suicide Screener	A standardized questionnaire for suicidality in minors	Not recommended for use with Latinx adolescents and may only be administered with English-speaking Latinx persons.
Beck Suicidal Ideation Scale	A standardized scale that screens for suicidality; there is no translation available in Spanish	The scale has serious limitations to validity when administered to Latinx children. Overall, not recommended for Latinx children.
Self-Harm Behavior Questionnaire	A screener for self-harm among minors; there is no translation available in Spanish	Recommended for English-speaking Latinx persons only.
Suicide Risk Inventory for Adolescents	Inventario de Riesgo Suicida para Adolescentes	A screener for suicidality in minors; available in English and Spanish	The scale is the only recommended suicidality measure of those presented here for Latinx Spanish-speakers given its availability in Spanish.
Acculturation		
Vancouver Index of Acculturation (VIA)	A 20-item multiethnic acculturation measure validated on culturally diverse samples, immigrants (Canada, Turkey, Italy, Arabs, and South Asians); it screens for orientation toward native and mainstream cultural values but excludes language	The scale has strong psychometric functions, but larger sample sizes are needed to replicate current validation studies with various immigrant groups. This scale may be best fitted for Canadian, Turkish, South Asian, and Arab immigrants.
Acculturation Rating Scale for Mexican Americans II	A bidimensional scale of acculturation for Mexican Americans; it measures Mexican and Anglo values with two subscales: Anglo Orientation Subscale (AOS) and the Mexican Orientation Subscale (MOS)	The scale can provide data of clinical utility to guide treatment planning decisions; the strong psychometric performance may be only limited to its screening ability in Mexican American adults. Other scales are recommended for caregivers and older adults, such as the Geriatric Acculturation Ratings Scale for Mexican Americans (G-ARSMA).

6

Troubleshooting

LINGUISTIC CONSIDERATIONS

Throughout the previous chapters of this book, we have highlighted that issues of language are intertwined with issues of validity and reliability in testing. While we have highlighted assessment measures available in Spanish, it is important to note that a Latinx client's preferred language may very well not be Spanish. Many Latinx persons in the United States speak Spanish only, many speak English only, many speak both, and many speak other languages including the native languages of Latin America. Also, speaking, listening, and writing skills may vary between English and Spanish in written assessments. Whether in assessment or psychotherapy cases, the initial cultural clinical interview must highlight the client's preferred language. Many times, as clinicians we get referrals from other medical providers, and our support staff are the first to collect this information and then decide clinician assignment and the client's language preference for intake paperwork. That first contact, whether by telephone or in person, is very important, and studies have identified that early contact between clients and clinic staff is essential to fostering a meaningful dialogue and future interactions (Akutsu & Chu, 2006). Living in a culturally diverse but predominantly Latinx community, English and Spanish intake documentation is readily available in our practice settings and many others. In settings like these, the clinician has some prior knowledge regarding a client's preferred language, and, as bilingual psychologists, we can navigate this process smoothly if the preferred language is one of those two. We have anecdotally found that ethnic and language matching facilitates this process, and extensive literature has supported the effects of client–provider matching by race/ethnicity and language (as well as matching by other variables like gender and sexual orientation; Karlsson, 2005; Maramba & Nagayama Hall, 2002). However, there are situations where Latinx clients do not speak English or Spanish. Having evaluated Latinx clients from other cultural or linguistic backgrounds, we have found the need and clinical utility of working with interpreters. Many clinicians may face similar situations working with Latinx and non-Latinx clients alike. Rather than making assumptions about a client's preferred language, cultural humility is demonstrated in asking the client their preferred language and making efforts to accommodate that preference.

WORKING WITH INTERPRETERS

Cultural humility and cultural competency will assist in making important clinical decisions with clients from different linguistic backgrounds and deciding when an interpreter is needed and who the interpreter should be. First, it is critical to understand the difference between *interpreters* and *translators*; these terms do not have the same meaning despite often being used interchangeably. In the clinical setting, it is best to use a competent interpreter who converts an oral message from one language to another. There are times when cultural concepts have no linguistic equivalence, and, at times like these, the interpreters' job is to convey the meaning and message with accuracy and completeness. A translator, in contrast, translates written text from one language to another. Both understand the cultural terms and idioms that provide meaning to the content, whether spoken or written. As mental health practitioners, it is critical to have interpreters available when rendering psychological services to those who do not speak your language. There are times when referring agencies and third parties provide a competent interpreter in person or a telehealth platform for interpreting. When they do not, it is the responsibility of the clinician to have a competent interpreter available for the session.

Mental health practitioners are responsible for ensuring that interpreters demonstrate competence, cultural sensitivity, and professionalism while providing a semantically accurate message translated from one language into another. It is equally recommended that clinicians take individual responsibility for making sure they themselves are skilled at working effectively with interpreters. At those times when clinicians do not speak the same language as their client, using an interpreter in psychological evaluations is more than simply having someone translate word for word the conversation between the client and the clinician. Interpreters bridge communication interactions between persons from different cultural and linguistic backgrounds. Accordingly, the communicative interaction taking place involves an intricate web of cultural communication styles, values, beliefs, and attitudes (Hwa-Froelich & Westby, 2003). It is critical that the interpreter can communicate this complex web of messages accurately and objectively.

Non-clinicians such as office managers or clerical staff are not appropriate personnel for the job of interpreter, given issues that may arise with them assuming multiple roles and because fluency in a language is not the same as competence in interpreting. Studies have demonstrated that untrained bilinguals might be able to maintain the accuracy of propositional content but be unable to recognize and accurately render the strategic use of discourse (Hale, Goodman-Delahunty, & Martschuk, 2019). Untrained bilinguals usually do not understand that they need to interpret the style and tone as well as the specific strategies used during questioning and interviewing. Many untrained bilinguals end up summarizing, rather than interpreting, content (Hale et al., 2019). It is, generally speaking, not appropriate to use family members and especially children as interpreters because doing so places them in a difficult role with their relative.

Mental health practitioners who use interpreters must obtain appropriate training, supervision, and consultation to adequately meet their ethical obligation of competence (American Psychological Association, 2010). Formal training should aim to assist clinicians in gaining insight into the nature of the services provided by interpreters and in enhancing their own competence in conducting psychological evaluations using an interpreter. They must acquire a greater level of reflection on their communication style and possess more clarity and thoughtfulness about language usage. If this is not possible due to various circumstances (e.g., time constraints when having to work with an interpreter unexpectedly, lack of training opportunities), clinicians should follow certain steps as outlined in this section. Likewise, clinicians should allocate sufficient time to consider the implications of working with an interpreter and consult with a more experienced colleague before their first evaluation using an interpreter. It is important to recognize and pay attention to the changes in in-room dynamics that the presence of an interpreter usually brings.

Mental health practitioners should identify the client's first language and find an interpreter who speaks this language or dialect and is, ideally, trained in the specific dialect used in the client's country of origin. Clinicians should make sure the interpreter is qualified, properly trained, and appropriate for the evaluation. The interpreter should not only be fluent in both languages but should understand the two different cultural contexts (Tribe & Raval, 2003). Furthermore, clinicians may match for gender and age between language interpreters and clients when possible as this could be helpful (Nijad, 2003).

Previous guidelines postulated by Searight and Armock (2013) identified a three-stage set of standards for clinicians to follow when using an interpreter. They proposed a pre-session meeting between the interpreter and clinician in advance of the session with the client, a discussion during the session with the client, and a post-session meeting between the clinician and interpreter. Taking this into account, clinicians should allow enough time for proper collaboration both before and during the evaluation. Equally, clinicians should be respectful to interpreters because they are important members of the team who make possible evaluations with linguistically diverse clients. Regarding the pre-session meeting, it is suggested that clinicians allocate 10–15 minutes to brief the interpreter about the nature of the evaluation and enable the interpreter to brief the clinician about any cultural issues that may have bearing on the evaluation. During this pre-session meeting, the clinician should instruct the interpreter to translate everything said, using first-person language and pronouns. Also, before the session starts, clinicians should consider the layout of the room and decide the positioning of chairs.

During the session, a clinician's behavior should change, to some extent, to accommodate interpreting. The clinician should start the session by introducing all participants and allow time for rapport-building before proceeding with the evaluation. In this context, clinicians should be mindful of issues of confidentiality and trust when working with individuals from diverse cultural backgrounds. Likewise, clinicians should strive to create a comfortable atmosphere where each member of the triad feels free to ask for clarification if anything is unclear. Searight and Armock (2013) advise clinicians to minimize eye contact with the interpreter and instead focus on the client. Doing so is harder than it sounds because often it feels as though one is speaking to the interpreter rather than the client! Clinicians should speak at an even pace in relatively short segments to allow for better interpretation. Also, clinicians should be aware that some words or idioms do not translate or do not have conceptual equivalents in other languages. By the same token, clinicians should avoid using complicated technical language or jargon.

Regarding the post-session, clinicians should allocate 10 minutes at the end of the evaluation to debrief the interpreter about the session. At this time, the clinician and the interpreter can provide feedback to each other and clarify any cultural or linguistic issues brought up by the session. Clinicians should be conscious of the well-being of the interpreter and the possibility that the interpreter may experience vicarious traumatization. Clinicians can use this post-evaluation meeting to offer support and process any emotional reactions that the interpreter may be having. Last, clinicians should consider the triadic relationship when interpreting the results from the evaluation and note the use of an interpreter in their report. For standardized testing, it is recommended to use measures that are specific to a client's language proficiency, as discussed previously.

BARRIERS TO TREATMENT AND ALLIANCE: DEALING WITH MICROAGGRESSIONS

Healthcare disparities have been present in the United States for decades, and, most recently, the COVID-19 pandemic has exposed deep disparities, with communities of color having been harmed disproportionately by this crisis (Garcini et al., 2021; Venta, Bick, & Bechelli, 2021). For example, African Americans are dying at nearly two times their national population share; in Arizona, American Indian death and case rates are five times the percentage of state population; in Washington, DC; Maryland; and Virginia, Latinx persons are 10 percent of the population yet make up a third of COVID-19 cases in that region (The Covidtracking Project, 2020). According to the Centers for Disease Control and Prevention (Cha & Cohen, 2020), Latinx persons are three times more likely to be uninsured and African Americans two times more likely to be uninsured than the White population.

Barriers to mental health treatment with ethnic minorities have also been present for many years. In a similar vein, Latinx as well as African American persons have substantially lower access to substance use treatment and mental health services (SAMSHA, 2020). Since the early 1980s epidemiological studies have documented the unmet mental health needs of Latinx persons (Cabassa et al., 2006). Epidemiological reviews have highlighted the complex interplay of structural, economic, psychiatric, and cultural variables that combine to play a role in access to mental health treatment in the Latinx community (Cabassa et al., 2006). The studies identified in Cabassas et al.'s (2006) review identified specific barriers that Latinx persons face in accessing mental healthcare, such as lack of health insurance, low acculturation levels, endorsing self-reliant attitudes, not knowing where to seek services, and high economic constraints. These factors have been repeatedly identified in scientific studies on healthcare disparities for decades, yet we continue to see inequity in mental healthcare today. According to the Office of the Surgeon General of the US (2001), mental healthcare disparities in the Latinx community have been severe, persistent, and well-documented throughout time. Latinx persons have less access to mental health services, are less likely to obtain care when needed, and are more likely to receive poor-quality care when treated (Chang, Natsuaki, & Chen, 2013: Maulik et al., 2014). Understanding Latinx mental health disparities requires an understanding and exploration of the cultural, social, legal, and practical barriers to care. Seeking and accessing treatment can be difficult and barriers include issues related to communication, lack of trust, provider's own biases, lack of insurance, and lack of representation in the workforce.

Turner et al. (2016) put forth a timely and pertinent conceptual model of treatment engagement that applies to culturally diverse groups and mental health services. The authors identified four barriers that ethnic minority groups encounter when help-seeking: accessibility, availability, appropriateness, and acceptability. For example, one of the first challenges for Latinx persons seeking mental health treatment is accessibility. The US mental health system is complex and can be difficult for even a knowledgeable person to navigate. A simple limitation for Latinx persons may be a lack of knowledge and awareness of services, as well as limited or no experience accessing and finding these services. Most mental health services are offered in settings separate from general medical care, and it is not always clear where and how to access these services (Guarnaccia et al., 2005). Research has demonstrated that having knowledge regarding where to find a provider significantly increases the likelihood of service utilization for Latinx persons (Turner et al., 2016). Relatedly, often, when service information is advertised it is not presented in Spanish and even less often in the other languages spoken by Latinx populations (Guarnaccia and Martinez, 2005). In addition, unfamiliarity with mental health services due to cultural differences can also increase wariness to accessing services because Latinx persons may not know what to expect from treatment, and, even if services are desired, the lack of mental health service coordination across healthcare settings and providers can still result in inappropriate services or lack of services completely (Chapa, 2004).

Immigration status is another prominent barrier contributing to accessibility to mental healthcare among the Latinx community (Livingston 2009). This barrier has intensified throughout the years, as many immigrant communities live in constant fear given the current anti-immigration policies and rhetoric in the United States. Families are afraid to leave their homes for fear of being deported and separated from their loved ones, let alone report these fears to a third-party provider who does not belong to their community. There has been a significant rise in deportations by US Customs and Immigration Enforcement (US Customs and Border Patrol, 2021), which contributes to these fears of deportation and may limit contact with healthcare providers.

Once mental health services are accessed by the few who are able to navigate the hurdles of accessibility, then availability of culturally sensitive mental health services and the appropriateness of such services and interventions are often problematic. A prominent issue in the field of mental health is the lack of psychological services delivered in the client's non-English native language, which significantly inhibits Latinx clients from seeking professional mental health services (Nielsen et al., 2016). Language barriers, as described earlier in this chapter, indeed limit the ability of some Latinx clients to communicate with monolingual English-speaking mental health clinicians. This difficulty plays a role in dissatisfaction with mental health services and may prompt premature termination. For example, a mental health practitioner trying to establish a therapeutic relationship with a client who has difficulty speaking English faces a challenging task, even if an interpreter is available. Many Latinx groups utilize English primarily in formal settings, such as in employment or legal settings, characterized by power differentials. As a result, the Latinx client may enter the assessment or therapy with an inclination to be subservient, which may contrast with the clinician's goal to establish a collaborative, open therapeutic relationship. Previous research has postulated that private and personal matters can be best expressed in one's native language and that clients can best express their feelings and emotions in their native tongue (Bailey et al., 2019; Venta, Muñoz, & Bailey, 2017). Thus, when clients with limited English proficiency are asked to communicate in English during a psychological assessment or therapy session, they may be unable to fully express their feelings and in fact may be misinterpreted and run the risk of being misdiagnosed (Venta et al., 2017). Having a culturally competent interpreter when a bilingual clinician is not readily available is strongly recommended.

Ethnic and Language Matching

In clinical settings, mental health practitioners will encounter some Latinx clients who prefer working with clinicians from a similar ethnic background, whereas other clients will not have such preference. In an early review of psychotherapeutic services conducted by Sue (1988), the effects of therapist ethnicity were mixed across studies, and Sue concluded that therapist ethnicity may not directly influence client preference, perceptions about therapist credibility, or treatment utilization patters. However, more recent research shows clients of color prefer therapists who are culturally similar to them, and research has illustrated benefits of ethnic matching on service utilization among Latinx populations (Turner et al., 2016). One assumption that has been in existence for many years is that White therapists matched with clients of color are not optimal. Sue (1988), however, challenged this notion, stating that ethnicity matching is a "distal" outcome in psychotherapy. Although he recognized the benefits of ethnic-matching, clients and therapist of the same ethnicity may have different cultural values and life experiences, and, conversely, they may share cultural values and life experiences but differ in ethnicity.

We have covered an array of barriers impeding Latinx persons in finding and utilizing mental healthcare. Barriers broadly cover issues related to the system structure, accessibility of care, the availability of cultural competent providers, the cultural appropriateness of treatment based on cultural conceptualizations of symptoms and mental illness, and the acceptability by the culture and larger society of utilizing mental health treatment. These obstacles include provider barriers, linguistic barriers, system barriers, financial barriers, and sociocultural barriers. These obstructions to mental health service utilization highlight potential areas for change that could improve the availability and access to services, which could ultimately improve utilization rates. Increasing the number of Spanish-speaking and culturally competent providers who are able to understand and respect the cultural values and conceptualizations of mental health of Latinx persons will be an important first step to engaging Latinx people in treatment. Healthcare reform has begun to address issues related to affordability, but this remains a pressing concern, particularly for Latinx immigrants. Given that Latinx persons are more likely to present in medical settings, integrating mental health referrals or providers into primary care settings can serve as one means to increasing service accessibility. Additionally, locating mental health services in the communities where Latinx persons live can both improve transportation issues as well as to help to destigmatize mental health treatment. With the emphasis placed on the family and potential childcare limitations, having options for childcare within agencies could greatly improve the feasibility of treatment utilization. Overall, the obstacles lying between Latinx persons and mental health treatment are plentiful and vast. Many have aimed to develop and implement best practices to engaging and working with the Latinx community, but it is clear that, without concerted effort and a commitment to structural changes to increase utilization, Latinx people will continue to remain underrepresented in our mental health system.

Dealing with Prejudice and Microaggressions

Microaggressions may occur during psychological assessments in therapeutic settings. Microaggressions may be made by clinicians and/or clients. Mental health practitioners will encounter patients who make prejudicial statements and display microaggression in the therapeutic setting and during psychological assessments.

Darland Wing Sue (2010) described racial microaggression as "everyday insults, indignities and demeaning messages sent to people of color" by individuals who are sometimes unaware of the offensive nature of their words or actions. Dr. Sue adds that microaggression can be broken down into three categories: microassaults, microinsults, and microinvalidations. *Microassaults* are more obvious and discriminatory behaviors, such as a client telling a racist joke or wearing a confederate flag in a session. *Microinsults* and *microinvalidations* are not as overt and tend to be unconscious and unintentional. For example, a well-intentioned perpetrator of a microinsult may believe they are being complimentary when they tell a Latinx client or mental health clinician they are "so articulate" or comment that "you do not have an accent." Microinvalidations, on the other hand, occur when people comment that they are "color blind" to racial differences, thus minimizing the struggles people of color have experienced over time, or they may simply state "racism does not exist anymore," thus minimizing current struggles.

These types of microaggressions can occur in a therapy or assessment session and they can come from the client or the clinician, often without the intention of hurting the other party. Nonetheless, as described in previous chapters, cultural humility can aid in the navigation of such experiences in the clinical setting and can serve as a buffer from such microaggressions coming from the clinician. However, microaggressions directed to mental health professionals can occur. Many people are uncomfortable and uneasy in acknowledging the delivery of microaggressions. Sue (2010) indicated that it is a scary thing to admit to having made a microaggression as doing so "assails their self-image of being good, moral, decent human beings to realize that maybe at an unconscious level they have biased thoughts, attitudes, and feelings that harm people of color." The perpetrator and even the recipient of microaggressions may try to brush off these statements and behaviors as not being a big deal, however, the cumulative effect of these interactions can be damaging to people of color's mental health and physical well-being (Nadal, 2014). Previous research has indicated that continuous exposure to these incidents is linked to depression and psychological trauma in addition to anxiety and high blood pressure (Franklin, 2019), among other health outcomes.

Knowing what to say can be difficult; some clinicians who adhere to social justice standards argue that these comments must be addressed, while others believe that they should be ignored (Mbroh et al., 2019). Mbroh et al. (2019) lay out ethical considerations involved in the decision-making process of the clinician when faced with such clients and situations. For example, the authors highlight that certain prejudicial beliefs are rooted in cultural and religious orientations, and ethical principles of psychology note we should respect that; however, the American Psychological Association (APA) states that psychologists "do not knowingly participate in or condone activities of others based on [patients'] prejudices." Moreover, the APA states that psychologists are expected to practice integrity by promoting accuracy, honesty, and truthfulness in the science, teaching, and practice of psychology. Thus, if clinicians and psychologists are aware that prejudicial beliefs harm their patients and that those beliefs may lead to prejudicial actions against others, then it is ethical for clinician to provide patients the tools needed to start questioning inaccurate prejudices and assumptions (Mbroh et al., 2019). The authors provide case scenarios that highlight ethical considerations and how clinicians should be proactive in their ethical decision-making. They also provide guidance regarding approaches to navigating these decisions. Ultimately, clinicians must thoroughly weigh the advantages and disadvantages of addressing patients' prejudicial beliefs and also engage in self-reflection to understand their own motives for addressing or not addressing prejudicial comments whenever possible. The process of self-reflection maybe difficult and overwhelming for some providers; thus, seeking consultation is critical. The authors end with an intervention scenario and highlight the importance of empathy, creating dissonance and highlighting benefit, and an invitation to explore.

TESTING WITH UNDOCUMENTED
CLIENTS: UNIQUE CONSIDERATIONS

Mental health practitioners will encounter adults, families, and children who are undocumented in various clinical settings. The results of psychological assessments with undocumented and immigrant groups can carry a large responsibility for the examiner because invalid, unsupported, or biased findings can lead to harmful consequences for the examinee, including in the context of immigration court if legal proceedings are ongoing. When working with a client who is undocumented, the consideration and integration of cultural factors as well as trauma-informed approaches discussed previously is essential, as described in previous chapters of this book. Relevant cultural factors include cultural response styles, cultural forms of emotional expression, and acculturation. Evaluators must consider the influence of these cultural factors on each aspect of the assessment of psychological functioning and psychopathology when making determinations regarding the examinee's mental health. Doing so includes giving consideration to cultural factors in the evaluation process, interpretation of data, and diagnosis.

As discussed in previous chapters, incorporating the use of culture and context-sensitive methodologies, as well as the use of assessment measures that are relevant and adapted for use with the target population, is critical when working with the undocumented client. The use of culture- and context-sensitive assessments in psychological evaluations is essential to facilitate understanding of the ways in which the immigration experience relates to or contributes to the immigrant's past and present physical and mental health distress, diminished well-being, and level of functioning.

It is important to include cultural factors in every part of the evaluation process when working with Latinx clients, but even more so when working with the undocumented client. Evaluators must familiarize themselves with psychometric theory and scientific methods that allow them to evaluate standard assessment instruments and methods by their scientific merits and value if they are to be used as evidence in legal procedures. Competency in all aspects of the assessment process, including psychological tests, goes beyond academic training to include familiarity with studies that extend the application of tests and critically evaluate their meaning in different populations.

The consideration of cultural factors applies during both the selection and administration of assessment measures. Steps must be taken to select assessment measures that are deemed appropriate for use with the specific cultural group of the client. In most cases, this means the measure has been developed and normed with the client's cultural group. In the absence of this, it is imperative to review relevant literature to ensure that the selected measure(s) have appropriate validity when used with the client's cultural group (Benuto, 2013). In the absence of literature to support of the use of the selected measure(s), attention must be given as to whether it is better to refrain from using the selected measure(s) or if steps should be taken to interpret the results of the measure(s) using a culturally informed interpretation strategy. Steps must also be taken to ensure that the administration of selected measure(s) is culturally informed as well. This includes being mindful of a client's reading and acculturation levels. For example, if the client has limited levels of formal education, it is often best to read test items to them. Therefore, it is important to allow additional time for test administration due to the added time that reading items to a client can add. Understanding an individuals' acculturation process and acculturative stress is necessary to best understand client presentation style, behavioral observations, and symptom presentation. For example, individuals with less contact with dominant US culture may require more cultural explanations, or translations may be necessary to ensure adequate understanding of test items.

Interpretation of the assessment data is another phase where a cultural lens must be applied, most importantly when the results stand in contrast to the clinical presentation. When a discrepancy of this type occurs, it is essential that the evaluator consider whether the discrepancy is related to the cultural limitations of an assessment measure(s) that may be contributing to inaccurate results. For instance, there is literature which suggests that difficulties understanding the Likert format of questionnaires can be common in the Latinx community (Butcher, Cabiya, Lucio, and Garrido, 2007). Consequently, a discrepancy between clinical presentation and Likert-based assessment results may be reflective of the clinical limitations of Likert scales and call into question the validity of the results. In these cases, use of clinical interview data in combination with collateral data from other mental health and medical providers may be the more culturally appropriate and valid assessment process.

As described in previous chapters, just as there are cultural variations in response style to assessment measures, there are cultural variations in emotional expression, also referred to as *cultural concepts of distress* (previously referred to as *culture-bound syndromes*) (American Psychiatric Association, 2013). Cultural concepts of distress refer to "ways that cultural groups experience, understand, and communicate suffering, behavioral problems, or troubling thoughts and emotions" (American Psychiatric Association, 2013, p. 758). The latest edition of the *Diagnostic and Statistical Manual of Mental Disorders* (DSM-5) emphasizes three different types of cultural concepts necessary to better understand and document distress among diverse populations (American Psychiatric Association, 2013). These include cultural syndromes, cultural idioms of distress, and cultural explanations or perceived causes.

The consideration and integration of contextual factors is essential. It is important for evaluators to consider the influence of contextual factors on each aspect of the assessment of psychological functioning and psychopathology when making determinations regarding the examinee's mental health. This includes consideration of contextual factors in the evaluation process, interpretation of data, and diagnosis. To adequately capture the effect of context on distress, evaluators should aim to document how context has influenced or is influencing the well-being and psychosocial functioning of the immigrant and the extent that context contributes to distress. Documentation is needed of how context contributes to behavioral, cognitive, and emotional responses experienced by immigrants when faced with situations of chronic and severe stress; this will avoid pathologizing the immigrant for reasons or influences over which the immigrant has little or no control (e.g., push factors in the country of origin that forced the migration process). In addition, documentation of the effect of contextual factors on all different aspects of the evaluation process is essential.

There are several sociodemographic and contextual factors that need to be assessed in psychological evaluations when working with the undocumented client. For instance, important contextual factors to consider and document include the possible detrimental effects on mental health, well-being, and psychosocial functioning of socioeconomic adversity (e.g., poverty, inadequate housing, hazardous living conditions, food insecurity), lack of or limited job and educational opportunities, exposure to hazardous environments or natural disasters, and loss or changes in objective and subjective social status at different stages of the immigration process, including pre-, during, and post-migration. Similarly, it is essential to document how difficulties and/or lack or limited access to needed services and resources, such as health and social services or legal protection, impact the immigrant's health and functioning. Also important to include in this type of psychological assessments is a description of how experiences of discrimination, marginalization, stigmatization, isolation, and/or exploitation may currently undermine an examinee's mental health and interpersonal interactions, as well as their effects over time given that these sources of distress have been found in research to impact mental health (Garcini et al., 2018). Moreover, migration-related losses that are important to assess and report include loss or changes in the immigrant's social support system (e.g., family separation, death of a distant loved one, disruption in social network); variations in self-image, including those attributed to changes in cultural values, practices, and/or traditions; loss of housing, land, and/or possessions; perceived loss of autonomy or freedom due to the examinee's immigration legal status; and loss or diminished physical health due to difficulties accessing healthcare and/or exposure to harsh living conditions and long-term toxic stressors. Likewise, the consideration of any cognitive and/or behavioral disabilities, learning difficulties, and/or functional impairments should also be documented in terms of how they have impacted the immigrant's life and migration journey, as well as their potential impact in the examinee's future functioning and quality of life. Additional contextual factors that are important to assess and document pertain to the immigrant's family environment and family dynamics. The migration process often changes a lot of the family dynamics that immigrants are most familiar with, thus increasing risk for distress and tension within the family system that may undermine the immigrant's mental health and functioning (e.g., changes in gender roles, family separation, disruption of intergenerational bonding).

Most recently, Mercado and colleagues (2022) published the first professional guidelines for psychological evaluations used in immigration proceedings. The guidelines include nine distinct professional standards highlighting competency, culture, contextual factors, psychometric theory, integration of intersecting identities, application of a trauma-informed framework, validity of the assessment, developmental framework with children, and the use of interpreters. The guidelines are aspirational in intent and intended to promote quality and consistency in the delivery of psychological immigration evaluations, as well as to provide a framework for conducting immigration evaluations.

Assessment of Undocumented Children

Psychological evaluations of undocumented immigrant children may be sought for a variety of reasons. One unique setting is immigration-related evaluation. Recent professional guidelines for immigration evaluations (Mercado et al., 2022) expand on the various types of psychological evaluations for adults and children and provide ethical standards for psychologists. Evaluations are often important to support asylum-seeking and other immigration relief petitions. These evaluations typically document the psychological impact of traumatic experiences to which children were exposed in their country of origin and during migration, as well as posttraumatic symptoms and resulting fears of returning home. This information helps establish an evidence base that can aid with legal determinations and identification of needed services. Additionally, the Office of Refugee Resettlement, Division of Unaccompanied Children Services (ORR/ DUCS), headed by the Department of Health and Human Services, often seeks evaluations for the children in their custody. These evaluations are not sought to answer a specific legal question but rather serve only clinical purposes. In this context, children may be referred for a psychological evaluation for various reasons, including diagnosis, safety concerns, or in the interest of treatment planning. It is important that evaluators understand the aim of the evaluation they are being asked to conduct, as the referral question should guide the instruments selected, the multiple informants sought for the evaluation, the framing of the report, and the type of recommendations included. Immigration evaluations may follow children for years within the immigration court system as well as outside of the court system, where they may access diverse services (e.g., special education services in school). It is essential that examiners are observant that their records do not cause harm both at the time of the evaluation and in the diverse contexts the child may eventually face (Evans & Graves, 2018).

A trauma-informed stance means that clinicians must be cognizant not to pathologize common experiences among immigrant youth. For example, substance use and other delinquent behaviors (e.g., theft, gang activity) are not uncommon among individuals seeking refuge in the United States and may even be considered a means of survival. These behaviors should not necessarily be interpreted as symptoms of externalizing behavior disorders. As such, an ever-growing foundation of cultural knowledge and respect for how contextual risk factors affect behavior is imperative when conducting such evaluations. In order to be developmentally sensitive, the evaluator must recognize that evaluations of children are best accomplished through the use of multiple informants, but the extent to which the child versus others can comment on the child's well-being changes across development (Howe, Goodman, & Cicchetti, 2008). Because immigrant children are often housed in a shelter or other caregiving arrangement, the evaluator must balance information sought from the clinician or legal guardian and the child in a developmentally sensitive manner. Children may have a limited understanding of who mental health practitioners are, what assessments are used for, and how the evaluation may affect them and their future. It is important to ensure that the minor's clinician has briefly explained the purpose of the evaluation to the child. Children may also be concerned that the evaluator works for Immigration and Customs Enforcement or other government organizations, that what the minor says will be used against them in immigration court, or that the evaluation will prevent unification with their family sponsor or a foster family. Both the minor and clinician or legal guardian should participate in discussing the minor's right to privacy, limits of confidentiality, procedure, role of the evaluator, aim of the evaluation, and purpose of the resulting assessment report in developmentally appropriate terms.

Cultural Adaptations

Psychologists must be mindful of the ways cultural and contextual adaptations can be used to ensure a culturally informed and relevant psychological evaluation process. Standard psychological assessment measures are not typically developed with the immigrant population. Often, they are not even developed for the population to which the examinee belongs. However, for an evaluation to be valid and reliable, the assessment process needs to use methodologies and measures that are sensitive to cultural and contextual variations in the examinee's response styles. Additionally, the process must capture the appropriate cultural constructs being evaluated so as not to distort the examinee's response style or responses as they relate to overall psychological functioning.

It is imperative that psychologists use cultural adaptations to ensure the psychological evaluation process is based on culturally and contextually appropriate practices, thereby ensuring the most accurate and valid information related to the client's psychological functioning. Bernal and Domenech Rodríguez (2012) describe how cultural adaptations can be used to ensure that evidence-based practices are culturally and contextually appropriate. These adaptations allow evaluators to gather important assessment data while being mindful of important cultural and contextual factors such as language, cultural values and constructs, worldviews, education level, socioeconomic status, immigration status, and acculturation. As discussed previously, such examples of cultural adaptations can include having the evaluator read items from questionnaires for clients who have limited formal education, who have lower reading abilities, or for whom a measure is not available in the client's preferred language. Cultural adaptations can also include changing Likert scales into yes or no questions or open-ended questions due to cultural variability with communication and worldviews (e.g., linear vs. circular) (Bernal & Doménech Rodriguez, 2012).

When cultural adaptations are made, it is important that all adaptations to standard administration are documented in the evaluation. The reason for the adaptation should be provided as well. Additionally, the evaluator must consider the ways in which changes to standard administration can impact scoring and interpretation of the results. For example, when reading items from a questionnaire, it is important to note whether the client appeared to demonstrate difficulties understanding the items and the response format (Likert or dichotomous). If limited difficulties were noted, then standard interpretation of the items may be appropriate. If, however, during the reading of a questionnaire, it appeared the client was confused by the question or the response format, a summary of the responses may be more appropriate.

Moreover, cultural adaptations can also be made by testing the client's limits with more culturally appropriate stimuli. For example, as discussed in Chapter 5, on cognitive tests that rely on visual images, it is important to consider the extent to which the client may have been exposed to the visual stimuli: Are the animals, drawings, and objects represented on the assessment stimuli consistent with animals, drawings, and objects the client could reasonably have been exposed to over the course of their lives? If not, consider completing the standard administration with the addition of more culturally relevant images to test the limits. In this case, score the standard administration and compare those scores to the more culturally relevant scores. If the scores overlap, then clinicians may have increased confidence in the results than if the scores are discrepant. In the latter situation, it is important to consider whether it is ethically appropriate to report assessment scores that are deemed to be an invalid representation of the client.

7

Future Directions in Psychological Assessment with Culturally Diverse Groups

As discussed in Chapter 4, progress is being made in examining and refining the psychometric properties of psychological instruments for use with Latinx persons. Still, this literature base remains relatively small, and, in most instances, psychometric studies of assessment tools fail to fully address measurement equivalence and method variance. Additional research in these areas is needed if practitioners are to have access to a full range of assessment instruments for use with Latinx clients. Relatedly, bilingualism complicates the assessment picture. While research on Spanish-English bilingualism is growing in the experimental and cognitive psychology fields, it has lagged behind in terms of psychological assessment (Bailey, Venta, & Langley, 2020). Little is known about how psychometric properties of instruments might be affected by degree of bilingualism, fluency, and acculturation to US norms and customs. These issues are particularly pronounced when considering semi-structured psychological instruments—commonly used in clinical practice—in which the language of assessment might obstruct significant clinical information (Venta, Muñoz, & Bailey, 2017).

RESEARCH ON THE ACCULTURATION AND ADAPTATION OF NEW WAVES OF IMMIGRANTS

Chapters 1–3 detailed some of the ways that recent immigrants are changing the landscape for mental health practice and research with Latinx groups in the United States. Briefly, recent decades have seen higher rates of migration from Central America's Northern Triangle (Guatemala, Honduras, and El Salvador) as well as greater migration of children and families. Emerging research suggests that trauma exposure (Venta, 2019; Venta & Mercado, 2019) and family separation (Venta et al., 2020) are more prevalent in recent waves of Latinx immigrants than in previous migratory groups and Latinx persons born in the United States. Recognizing that trauma and separation can affect health (Mercado, Venta, Henderson, & Pimentel, 2019) and acculturation after migration (Venta, 2020), it will be essential for future research to focus on risk and protective factors that are applicable to recent waves of immigrant in order to refine psychological instruments for use in that group. Indeed, previous notions of the Hispanic Health Paradox may need to be revised as we gain scientific knowledge about recent immigrant groups.

Recognition of within-group variability among Latinx persons. As we summarized earlier in the book, Latinx people are a diverse group: some are immigrants and some are not; some are fluent in English, Spanish, or both and some are fluent in only one or neither; some adhere to traditional cultural values like *machismo* and *marianismo*, and some find these cultural views foreign; some came to the United States by choice and knew prosperity from their arrival, and some struggled to adapt to their new country, having been forcibly displaced from their home countries; some are from just the other side of the southern US border, and some are from thousands of miles away. These are just some of the many variables that produce within-group heterogeneity and variability among Latinx persons living in the United States. Psychological research has done very little to unpack how this variability might affect psychological testing. This type of research has lagged behind the other advances included in this book, partially because it requires large sample sizes that allow examination of within-group variability. Research with Latinx persons often utilizes samples that are small or moderately sized, powered only to examine basic questions about Latinx versus non-Latinx group differences (and, at time, underpowered for even those analyses). Collaboration among researchers interested in Latinx persons is essential for developing large-scale studies in which attention can be paid to the aforementioned areas of heterogeneity as well as many other facets of diversity, including intersectionality with gender identity, sexual orientation, and other aspects of identity. Associations like the National Latinx Psychological Association and their flagship journal, the *Journal of Latinx Psychology*, are promising avenues for facilitating the scholarly collaboration needed for advancing research on within-group variability among Latinx people.

Increased consideration of clinical samples in research with Latinx persons. To enhance the clinical utility of empirical research with Latinx persons, particularly assessment research, samples must also include individuals demonstrating severe symptoms, including those seeking outpatient clinical care and those in inpatient facilities. While research with Latinx college students and community dwellers has advanced our knowledge of how bilingualism, acculturation, and Latinx cultural values relate to mental health and assessment, these variables are rarely considered in studies of serious mental illness or in samples experiencing severe psychological symptoms more generally. As a result, clinical recommendations made for Latinx persons are often based on anecdotal reports because no data are available (e.g., Muñoz & Venta, 2019) or make use of community-based research. In the future, research with clinical samples must include variables known to be relevant to the mental health of Latinx persons (e.g., acculturation), and assessment research must include Latinx participants at the severe end of psychopathology spectra.

Expanding training and evidence-based practices. Another area of future consideration includes expanding evidenced-based practices with immigrant groups. Currently, there are no specific evidenced-based clinical interventions for specific immigrant groups. Clinical research highlighting best practices are needed. In addition, there is a dire need for trauma-informed systems when working with Latinx groups including immigrants. Also, dissemination of evidenced-based information using non-traditional sources with this population is important and another way of reaching these clients.

A CALL TO ACTION

According to Haile Selassie, "Throughout history it has been the inaction of those who could have acted, the indifference of those who should have known better, the silence of the voice of justice when it mattered most, that have made it possible for [harm] to triumph." Advocacy is one of the main avenues that can help to support, bolster, and strengthen communities of color like Latinx and immigrant communities. Advocacy can spotlight the unjust inequities faced by so many and serve as a catalyst to prompt necessary action. The collective voice of strategic advocacy initiatives has the power to move mountains. In addition, the integration of advocacy into one's professional identity may serve to protect against burnout as providers are able to engage in meaningful change. Garcini et al. (2021) provides six recommendations for psychologists to help guide social change.

1. *Support efforts aimed at terminating harsh rhetoric and exclusionary and discriminatory policies, inhumane treatment, and violations of human rights.* The negative impact of anti-immigration policy has been studied and concluded to be harmful (Cervantes & Walker, 2017; Wood, 2018). Policymakers and providers need to move away from this approach to create opportunities for engaging in respectful dialogue about immigration that can help us find practical and proactive solutions based on evidence, rather than reinforce anti-immigrant rhetoric and practices. Finding effective ways of communicating different perspectives and talking to people about controversial immigration issues must be a priority. This requires building avenues for learning about our immigrant communities and disseminating information that can help debunk existing stereotypes. For example, finding and disseminating stories of overcoming and success among immigrant communities can serve to counter those that present the community as weak, helpless, or dependent.

2. *Support immigrant efforts, whether directly or indirectly.* Everyone has access to unique platforms depending on their areas of expertise,

access to resources, and employment settings. Whether in academia, medical centers, private or community organizations, leadership boards, or even in local neighborhoods, people can use their access to such platforms to advocate for change and to end the stereotyping of at-risk immigrants. In reminding others about core American values such as morality and humanitarianism, individuals can invite others to dialogue that can foster social change. Indeed, research provides evidence for curriculum and training that may be delivered within institutions and organizations to educate and improve attitudes toward immigrants (Cadenas et al., 2018). Moreover, as health professionals, we may use our background and skills to educate, serve, and inform the needs of immigrant organizations or provide pro bono services for at-risk immigrants. Professionals can also join the movement for change, particularly at the intersection of immigrant rights and racial justice. Examples of how providers may support immigrants include advocating for safe spaces and specialized programs, such as the creation of resources and information centers (Cisneros & Rivarola, 2020). While these centers have been pioneered in higher education, similar programs may be developed within K-12 schools, healthcare delivery systems, and community organizations, as well as within advocacy organizations.

3. *Contribute to building a workforce equipped to meet the need of at-risk immigrants.* Regardless of field of study, professionals can support the training efforts of students, colleagues, or younger professionals who may be interested in working with immigrant communities as well as support immigrants seeking to develop the education and skills necessary for career advancement. This requires that providers expand their knowledge base and develop competencies in this area. Seeds need to be planted to build a workforce of future professionals and researchers equipped to work with immigrant communities and one that involves community partners and members. Cadenas et al. (2018) provides specific recommendations for how providers may advocate for workforce development of those serving immigrants and immigrant communities themselves.

4. *Assist in research efforts.* Knowledge about the complex needs of undocumented immigrants is limited. This information is essential to inform interventions, advocacy, and, most importantly, policy efforts. Efforts to build interdisciplinary collaborations to advance research in this area are much needed, along with advocacy for funding to support research and clinical efforts. Moreover, the reasons underlying the ambivalence and mistrust of research exhibited by communities of color has to be recognized and addressed. Building partnership and collaborations is important. Members of immigrant communities should be fully informed of the purpose of the research and the risks and benefits associated with their participation. Students and professionals leading these efforts must be educated on relevant historical events and

find ways to honor and respond to the narratives of the community they seek to study.

5. *Serve as a role model in everyday life.* Another way to become advocates is by setting an example for others. It is important to embody humility in working and interacting with at-risk immigrants. There is scholarship that specifically details how to develop the cultural and contextual competency needed to work with vulnerable communities, including immigrants (Lund & Lee, 2015). Indeed, it is possible to structure learning opportunities for current providers and providers-in-training to develop humility as a skill and mindset that will aid them in competently serving immigrant communities.

6. *Seek opportunities to build community alliances.* Immigrant communities often engage with numerous organizations and systems. In addition to healthcare providers, schools, faith-based institutions, and churches can represent natural partners in this work (e.g., Parra-Cardona et al., 2016). Providers should reach out to and familiarize themselves with available resources and lead the development of partnerships that will meet the varied needs of immigrants.

Last, another way that psychologists and mental health clinicians can make a difference is being active members and future leaders of psychological and/or mental health associations. Being present and sitting at the table where important decisions are made for our profession is critical in making meaningful change in our profession.

CONCLUSION

This book is intended to be a resource for psychologists and mental health professionals when working with Latinx clients in the psychological assessment context. Far too many times, we have seen psychological evaluations that have misdiagnosed clients and have used psychological batteries that were questionable. We hope this book is used by clinicians to further hone their skills in psychological assessment when working with Latinx populations. It is critical that clinicians highlight culture in the assessment process and include culture in the case formulation, which will guide a culturally informed framework that will then lead to careful selection of psychological batteries and a sound case conceptualization that will further provide rich information needed for an individualized treatment plan and culturally responsive clinical recommendations. The role of cultural humility in the psychological assessment context is also critical. It is also important to understand that seeking consultation is recommended when needed, and a referral to a psychologists or mental health practitioners with extensive experience with Latinx populations may be warranted. There are many opportunities for clinical trainings that address culture and diversity at the state and national levels, including the American Psychological Association's innovative workshops and professional development opportunities that teach how to effectively work with Latinx and immigrant communities (Cadenas et al., 2022). It is essential that mental health practitioners build cultural competency in psychological assessment to effectively collaborate and work with Latinx populations. It is the responsibility of mental health professionals to assure that clinical assessments adhere to ethical standards and apply culturally informed practices.

REFERENCES

Abate, A., Bailey, C., & Venta, A. (2022). Attachment and social support in Latinx young adults: Investigating the moderating role of familismo. *Journal of Cross-Cultural Psychology, 53*(3–4), 327–343. https://doi.org/10.1080/14616734.2019.1664604

Acevedo-Garcia D., & Bates L. M. (2008). Latino health paradoxes: Empirical evidence, explanations, future research, and implications. In H. Rodríguez, R. Sáenz, C. Menjívar (Eds.), *Latinas/os in the United States: Changing the face of América.* Boston, MA: Springer. https://doi.org/10.1007/978-0-387-71943-6_7

Acevedo-Polakovich, I. D., Reynaga-Abiko, G., Garriott, P. O., Derefinko, K. J., Wimsatt, M. K., Gudonis, L. C., & Brown, T. L. (2007). Beyond instrument selection: Cultural considerations in the psychological assessment of US Latinas/os. *Professional Psychology: Research and Practice, 38*(4), 375. https://doi.org/10.1037/0735-7028.38.4.375

Achenbach, T. M., & Rescorla, L. A. (2000). *Manual for the ASEBA preschool forms and profiles* (Vol. 30). Burlington, VT: University of Vermont, Research center for children, youth, & families.

Achenbach, T. M. (1999). The Child Behavior Checklist and related instruments. In M. E. Maruish (Ed.), *The use of psychological testing for treatment planning and outcome assessment* (pp. 429–466). New York: Lawrence Erlbaum.

AERA, APA, & NCME. (1999). *The standards for educational and psychological testing.* Washington, DC: AERA.

Aggarwal, N. K, Nicasio, A. V., DeSilva, R., Boiler, M., & Lewis-Fernandez, R. (2013). Barriers to implementing the DSM5 Cultural Formulation Interview: A qualitative study. *Cultural Medical Psychiatry, 37*, 505–533.

Akutsu, P. D., & Chu, J. P. (2006). Clinical problems that initiate professional help-seeking behaviors from asian americans. *Professional Psychology: Research and Practice, 37*(4), 407. https://doi.org/10.1037/0735-7028.37.4.407

Alamilla, S. G., & Wojcik, J. V. (2013). Assessing for personality disorders in the Hispanic client. In L. T. Benuto (Ed.), *Guide to psychological assessment with Hispanics* (pp. 215–241). New York: Springer.

Alba, R. D., & Nee, V. (2005). Assimilation and contemporary immigration. *Remaking the American Mainstream, 2*, 215–270.

Alegría, M., Canino, G., Shrout, P. E., Woo, M., Duan, N., Vila, D., . . . Meng, X. L. (2008). Prevalence of mental illness in immigrant and non-immigrant U.S. Latino groups. *The American Journal of Psychiatry, 165*(3), 359–369. https://doi.org/10.1176/appi.ajp.2007.07040704

Alegria, M., Nakash, O., & NeMoyer, A. (2018). Increasing equity in access to mental healthcare: A critical first step in improving service quality. *World Psychiatry, 17*(1), 43–44.

Allen, B., Cisneros, E. M., & Tellez, A. (2015). The children left behind: The impact of parental deportation on mental health. *Journal of Child and Family Studies, 24*(2), 386–392.

American Psychiatric Association (1994*). Diagnostic and statistical manual of mental disorders* (4th ed.). Washington, DC: Author.

American Psychiatric Association. (2013). *Diagnostic and statistical manual of mental disorders* (5th ed.). Washington, DC: American Psychiatric Association Publishing.

American Psychiatric Association. (2019). Structured Clinical Interview for the DSM5. Retrieved from https://www.appi.org/products/structured-clinical-interv iew-for-dsm-5-scid-5

American Psychological Association. (2010). Ethical principles of psychologists and code of conduct (2002, Amended June 1, 2010). http://www.apa.org/ethics/code/ index.aspx

American Psychological Association. (2017). Ethical principles of psychologists and code of conduct (2002, amended effective June 1, 2010, and January 1, 2017). https:// www.apa.org/ethics/code/index.aspx

American Psychological Association. (2017). Multicultural guidelines: An ecological approach to context, identity, and intersectionality, 2017. Retrieved from http://www. apa.org/about/policy/multiculturalguidelines.Aspx

American Psychological Association. (2019). APA Guidelines on Race and Ethnicity in Psychology 2019. Retrieved from https://www.apa.org/about/policy/guidelines-race-ethnicity.pdf

American Psychological Association. (2019). Deep Poverty Initiative. https://www.apa. org/about/governance/president/deep-poverty-initiative.

Arciniega, G. M., Anderson, T. C., Tovar-Blank, Z. G., & Tracey, T. J. G. (2008). Toward a fuller conception of machismo: Development of a traditional Machismo and Caballerismo Scale. *Journal of Counseling Psychology, 55*(1), 19–33. https://doi.org/ 10.1037/0022-0167.55.1.19

Ávila-Espada, A. (2000). Objective scoring for the TAT. In R. H. Dana (Ed.), *Handbook of cross-cultural and multicultural personality assessment* (pp. 465–480). Mahwah, NJ: Erlbaum.

Azocar, F., Areán, P., Miranda, J., & Muñoz, R. F. (2001). Differential item functioning in a Spanish translation of the Beck Depression Inventory. *Journal of Clinical Psychology, 57*(3), 355–365. https://doi.org/10.1002/jclp.1017

Bailey, C., McIntyre, E., Arreola, A., & Venta, A. (2019). What are we missing? How language impacts trauma narratives. *Journal of Child & Adolescent Trauma, 13*(2), 153–161.

Báguena, M. J., Villarroya, E., Belena, A., Díaz, A., Roldan, C., & Reig, R. (2001). Propiedades psicométricas de la versión española de la Escala Revisada de Impacto del Estresor (EIE-R). *Análisis Y Modificación de Conducta, 27*(114), 581–604.

Bailey, C., Venta, A., & Langley, H. (2020). The bilingual [dis]advantage. *Language and Cognition, 12*(2), 225–281. https://doi.org/10.1017/langcog.2019.43

Bialystok, E., Craik, F., & Luk, G. (2008). Cognitive control and lexical access in younger and older bilinguals. *Journal of Experimental Psychology: Learning, Memory, and Cognition, 34*, 859–873. http://dx.doi.org/10.1037/0278-7393.34.4.859

Beehler, S., Birman, D., & Campbell, R. (2012). The effectiveness of cultural adjustment and trauma services (CATS): Generating practice-based evidence on a comprehensive, school-based mental health intervention for immigrant youth. *American Journal of Community Psychology, 50*(1), 155–168.

Ben-Porath, Y., & Tellegen, A. (2008). *Minnesota Multiphasic Personality Inventory-2-Restructured Form (MMPI-2-RF)* [Database record]. APA PsycTests. https://doi.org/10.1037/t15121-000

Benuto, L. T. (2013). *Guide to psychological assessment with Hispanics.* Springer.

Bernal, G. E., & Domenech Rodríguez, M. M. (2012). *Cultural adaptations: Tools for evidence-based practice with diverse populations.* American Psychological Association.

Bird, H. R. (1996). Epidemiology of childhood disorders in a cross-cultural context. *Journal of Child Psychology and Psychiatry, and Allied Disciplines, 37*(1), 35–49. https://doi.org/10.1111/j.1469-7610.1996.tb01379.x

Boscán, D. C., Penn, N. E., Velasquez, R. J., Reimann, J., Gomez, N., Guzman, M., . . . De Romero, M. C. (2000). MMPI-2 profiles of Colombian, Mexican, and Venezuelan university students. *Psychological Reports, 87*(1), 107–110.

Bourke, D. H. (2014). *Immigration: Tough questions, direct answers.* Downers Grove, IL: InterVarsity Press.

Borum, R., Bartel, P., & Forth, A. (2006). *Manual for the Structured Assessment for Violence Risk in Youth (SAVRY).* Odessa, FL: Psychological Assessment Resources.

Breland-Noble, A. M. (2013). The impact of skin color on mental health and behavioral health in African-American and Latina adolescent girls: A review of the literature. In R. E. Hall (Ed.), *The melanin millennium: Skin color as 21st century international discourse* (pp. 219–229). Dordrecht: Springer Science + Business Media.

Breslau, J., Borges, G., Tancredi, D., Saito, N., Kravitz, R., Hinton, L., . . . Aguilar-Gaxiola, S. (2011). Migration from Mexico to the United States and subsequent risk for depressive and anxiety disorders: A cross-national study. *Archives of general psychiatry, 68*(4), 428–433. https://doi.org/10.1001/archgenpsychiatry.2011.21

Bronfenbrenner, U. (1992). Ecological systems theory. In R. Vasta (Ed.), *Six theories of child development: Revised formulations and current issues* (pp. 187–249). London: Jessica Kingsley Publishers.

Buhs, E. S., McGinley, M., & Toland, M. D. (2010). Overt and relational victimization in Latinos and European Americans: Measurement equivalence across ethnicity, gender, and grade level in early adolescent groups. *The Journal of Early Adolescence, 30*(1), 171–197. https://doi.org/10.1177/0272431609350923

Bulut, E., & Gayman, M. D. (2015). Acculturation and self-rated mental health among Latino and Asian immigrants in the United States: A latent class analysis. *Journal of Immigrant and Minority Health, 18*(4), 836–849. https://doi.org/10.1007/s10903-015-0258-1

Butcher, J. N., Cabiya, J., Lucio, E., & Garrido, M. (2007). *Assessing Hispanic clients using the MMPI-2 and MMPI-A.* American Psychological Association. https://doi.org/10.1037/11585-000

Butcher, J. N., Cabiya, J., Lucio, E., & Garrido, M. (2007). The international assessment context: Spanish language adaptations of the MMPI, MMPI-2, and MMPI-A. In J. N. Butcher, J. Cabiya, E. Lucio, & M. Garrido (Eds.), *Assessing Hispanic clients using the MMPI-2 and MMPI-A* (pp. 25–54). American Psychological Association.

Byrne, B. M., Shavelson, R. J., & Muthén, B. (1989). Testing for the equivalence of factor covariance and mean structures: The issue of partial measurement invariance. *Psychological Bulletin, 105*(3), 456–466. https://doi.org/10.1037/0033-2909.105.3.456

Cabassa, L. J., Zayas, L. H., & Hansen, M. C. (2006). Latino adults' access to mental health care: A review of epidemiological studies. *Administration and Policy in Mental Health and Mental Health Services Research, 33*(3), 316–330. https://doi.org/10.1007/s10488-006-0040-8

Cabiya, J. J., Chavira, D. A., Gomez Jr, F. C., Lucio, E., Castellanos, J., & Velasquez, R. J. (2000). MMPI-2 scores of Puerto Rican, Mexican, and US Latino college students: A research note. *Psychological Reports, 87*(1), 266–268.

Cadenas, G. A., Neimeyer, G., Suro, B., Minero, L. P., Campos, L., Garcini, L. M., . . . Domenech Rodríguez, M. M. (2022). Developing cultural competency for providing psychological services with immigrant populations: A cross-level training curriculum. *Training and Education in Professional Psychology, 16*(2), 121. https://doi.org/10.1037/tep0000380

Cadenas, G. A., Cisneros, J., Todd, N. R., & Spanierman, L. B. (2018). DREAMzone: Testing two vicarious contact interventions to improve attitudes toward undocumented immigrants. *Journal of Diversity in Higher Education, 11*(3), 295–308. https://doi.org/10.1037/dhe0000055

Caldwell, A., Couture, A., & Nowotny, H. (2008). *Closing the mental health gap: Eliminating disparities in treatment for Latinos.* Kansas City, MO: Mattie Rhodes Center.

Caplan, S. (2007). Latinos, acculturation, and acculturative stress: A dimensional concept analysis. *Policy, Politics, & Nursing Practice, 8*(2), 93–106.

Cardemil, E. V. (2010). Cultural adaptations to empirically supported treatments: A research agenda. *The Scientific Review of Mental Health Practice, 7*(2), 8–21.

Carlos, J., & Gonzalez, S. (2015). Using Pruebas Publicadas en Espanol to Enhance Test Selection. In K. F. Geisinger (Ed.), *Psychological testing of Hispanics: Clinical, cultural, and intellectual issues* (2nd ed., pp. 11–28). American Psychological Association: Washington, DC.

Casas, J. M., Furlong, M. J., Alvarez, M., & Wood, M. (1998). Que Dice? Initial Analyses Examining Three Spanish Translations of the CBCL. Retrieved from https://eric.ed.gov/?id=ED432866

Carlson, S. M., & Meltzoff, A. N. (2008). Bilingual experience and executive functioning in young children. *Developmental Science, 11*, 282–298. http://dx.doi.org/10.1111/j.1467-7687.2008.00675.x

Casas, J. M. (2017). *Handbook of multicultural counseling* (4th ed.). SAGE Publications, Inc.

Casas, J. M., & Cabrera, A. P. (2011). Latino/a Immigration: Actions and outcomes based on perceptions and emotions or facts? *Hispanic Journal of Behavioral Sciences, 33*(3), 283–303.

Castaneda, H., Holmes, S. M., Madrigal, D. S., De Trinidad Young, M. E., Beyeler, N., & Quesasa, J. (2015). Immigration as a social determinant of health. *Annual Review of Puublic Health, 36*, 375–392.

Castillo, L. G., Perez, F. V., Castillo, R., & Ghoshed, M. (2010). Construction and initial validation of the Marianismo Beliefs Scale. *Counseling Psychology Quarterly, 23*(2), 163–175. https://doi.org/10.1080/09515071003776036

Cervantes, W., & Walker, C. (2017). Five reasons Trump's immigration orders harm children. *Washington, DC: Center for Law and Social Policy*, 1–8.

Cha, A. E., & Cohen, R. A. (2020). *Reasons for being uninsured among adults aged 18–64 in the United States, 2019. NCHS Data Brief, no 382.* Hyattsville, MD: National Center for Health Statistics.

Chang, J., Natsuaki, M. N., & Chen, C. N. (2013). The importance of family factors and generation status: mental health service use among Latino and Asian Americans. *Cultural Diversity and Ethnic Minority Psychology, 19*(3), 236. https://doi.org/10.1037/a0032901

Chapa, T. (2004). *Mental health services in primary care settings for racial and ethnic minority populations.* Department of Health & Human Services, Office of Minority Health.

Cisneros, J., & Rivarola, A. R. R. (2020). Undocumented student resource centers. *Journal of College Student Development, 61*(5), 658–662. https://doi.org/10.1353/csd.2020.0064

Clahsen, H., & Felser, C. (2006). Grammatical processing in language learners. *Applied Psycholinguistics, 27*(1), 3–42. doi:10.1017/S0142716406060024

Clark, L., Bunik, M., & Johnson, S. (2010). Research opportunities with Curanderos to address childhood overweight in Latino families. *Qualitative Health Research, 20*(1), 4–14. doi:10.1177/1049732309355285

Clauss-Ehlers, C. S., Chiriboga, D. A., Hunter, S. J., Roysircar, G., & Tummala-Narra, P. (2019). APA multicultural guidelines executive summary: Ecological approach to context, identity, and intersectionality. *American Psychologist, 74*(2), 232–244. https://doi.org/10.1037/amp0000382

Council of National Psychological Associations for the Advancement of Ethnic Minority Interests. (2016). *Testing and assessment with persons & communities of color.* Washington, DC: American Psychological Association. Retrieved from https://www.apa.org/pi/oema

Council of Social Work Education. (2022). Center for Diversity and Social & Economic Justice. Retrieved from https://www.cswe.org/Centers-Initiatives/Centers/Center-for-Diversity/Curriculum-Resources/EPAS-Curricular-Guide-on-Diversity-and-Social-Ec

Cuéllar, I. (1998). Cross-cultural clinical psychological assessment of Hispanic Americans. *Journal of Personality Assessment, 70*(1), 71–86. https://doi.org/10.1207/s15327752jpa7001_5

Cuellar, I., Arnold, B., & Maldonado, R. (1995). Acculturation Rating Scale for Mexican Americans-II: A revision of the original ARSMA scale. *Hispanic Journal of Behavioral Sciences, 17*(3), 275–304. https://doi.org/10.1177/07399863950173001

Cuevas, J. L., & Osterich, H. (1990). Cross-cultural evaluation of the booklet version of the Category Test. *International Journal of Clinical Neuropsychology, 12*, 187–190.

Curiel, R. E., Hernández-Cardenache, R., Giraldo, N., Rosado, M., Restrepo, L., Raffo, A., Lavado, M., Santos, J., & Whitt, N. M. (2016). A compendium of neuropsychological measures for Hispanics in the United States. In F. R. Ferraro (Ed.), *Minority and cross-cultural aspects of neuropsychological assessment: Enduring and emerging trends* (pp. 471–514). Taylor & Francis.

Dana, R. H. (1993). *Multicultural assessment perspectives for professional psychology.* Allyn & Bacon.

Dana, R. H. (1998). Cultural identity assessment of culturally diverse groups: 1997. *Journal of Personality Assessment, 70*(1), 1–16. https://doi.org/10.1207/s15327752jpa7001_1

Dana R. H. (2013). Culture and Methodology in Personality Assessment. In F. A. Paniagua, & A. M. Yamada (Eds.), *Handbook of multicultural mental health: Assessment and treatment of diverse populations* (2nd ed., pp. 205–224). San Diego: Elsevier. http://dx.doi.org/10.1016/B978-0-12-394420-7.00011-4

Dana, R. H. (2015). A personality approach to testing Hispanics. In K. F. Geisinger (Ed.), *Psychological Testing of Hispanics: Clinical, Cultural, and Intellectual Issues* (2nd ed., pp. 189–214), Washington, DC: American Psychological Association.

Dana, R. H. (1999). Cross-cultural-multicultural use of the Thematic Apperception Test. In L. Gieser & M. I. Stein (Eds.), *Evocative images: The Thematic Apperception Test and the art of projection* (pp. 177–190). American Psychological Association.

Diaz-Rico, L. T., & Weed, K. Z. (2006). *The cross-cultural language and academic development handbook: A complete K-12 reference guide* (3rd ed.). Boston: Pearson.

Dunnigan, T., McNall, M., & Mortimer, J. T. (1993). The problem of metaphorical nonequivalence in cross-cultural survey research: Comparing the mental health statuses of Hmong refugee and general population adolescents. *Journal of Cross-Cultural Psychology, 24*(3), 344–365. https://doi.org/10.1177/0022022193243005

Eaton, W. W., Smith, C., Ybarra, M., Muntaner, C., & Tien, A. (2004). Center for Epidemiologic Studies Depression Scale: Review and Revision (CESD and CESD-R). In M. E. Maruish (Ed.), *The use of psychological testing for treatment planning and outcomes assessment: Instruments for adults* (pp. 363–377). Marwah: Lawrence Erlbaum Associates Publishers.

Edwards, R. G., & Beiser, M. (1994). Southeast Asian refugee youth in Canada: The determinants of competence and successful coping. *Canada's Mental Health, 42*(1), 1–5.

Edwards, L. M., & Cardemil, E. V. (2015). Clinical approaches to assessing cultural values among Latinos. In K. F. Geisinger (Ed.), *Psychological testing of Hispanics: Clinical, cultural, and intellectual issues* (pp. 215–236). American Psychological Association. https://doi.org/10.1037/14668-012

Ehntholt, K. A., & Yule, W. (2006). Practitioner review: Assessment and treatment of refugee children and adolescents who have experienced war-related trauma. *Journal of Child Psychology and Psychiatry, and Allied Disciplines, 47*(12), 1197–1210. https://doi.org/10.1111/j.1469-7610.2006.01638.x

Elliott, C. D. (2012). *Administration and technical manual for the Differential Abilities Scale: Second edition. Early years Spanish supplement*. San Antonio: Pearson.

Ellison, J., Jandorf, L., & Duhamel, K. (2011). Assessment of the Short Acculturation Scale for Hispanics (SASH) among low-income, immigrant Hispanics. *Journal of Cancer Education: The Official Journal of the American Association for Cancer Education, 26*(3), 478–483. https://doi.org/10.1007/s13187-011-0233-z

Ephraim, D., Söchting, I., & Marica, J. E. (1997). Cultural norms for TAT narratives in psychological practice and research: Illustrative studies. *Rorschachiana, 22*(1), 13–37.

Ephraim, D. (2000). A psychocultural approach to TAT scoring and interpretation. *Handbook of cross-cultural and multicultural personality assessment* (pp. 427–445). Lawrence Erlbaum Associates.

Erolin, K. S., Wieling, E., & Parra, R. E. A. (2014). Family violence exposure and associated risk factors for child PTSD in a Mexican sample. *Child Abuse & Neglect, 38*(6), 1011–1022.

Estrada, A. R., & Smith, S. R. (2019). An exploration of Latina/o respondent scores on the Personality Assessment Inventory. *Current Psychology, 38*(3), 782–791.

Evans, C., & Graves, K. (2018). Trauma among children and legal implications. *Cogent Social Sciences, 4*(1), 1546791. https://doi.org/10.1080/23311886.2018.1546791

Fazel, M., Reed, R. V., Panter-Brick, C., & Stein, A. (2012). Mental health of displaced and refugee children resettled in high-income countries: Risk and protective factors. *Lancet (London, England), 379*(9812), 266–282. https://doi.org/10.1016/S0140-6736(11)60051-2

Federal Strategic Action Plan on Services for Victims of Human Trafficking in the United States. (2014). *Federal Strategic Action Plan on Services for Victims of Human Trafficking in the United States 2013–2017*. Retrieved from https://ovc.ojp.gov/sites/g/files/xyckuh226/files/media/document/FederalHumanTraffickingStrategicPlan.pdf

Fenollar-Cortes, J., & Watkins, M. W. (2019). Construct validity of the Spanish version of the WISCV Spain. *International Journal of School and Educational Psychology, 7*(3), 150–164.

Fernandez, K., Boccaccini, M. T., & Noland, R. M. (2007). Professionally responsible test selection for Spanish-speaking clients: A four-step approach for identifying and selecting translated tests. *Professional Psychology: Research and Practice, 38*(4), 363–374. https://doi.org/10.1037/0735-7028.38.4.363

Fernandez, K., Boccaccini, M. T., & Noland, R. M. (2008). Detecting over- and underreporting of psychopathology with the Spanish-language Personality Assessment Inventory: Findings from a simulation study with bilingual speakers. *Psychological Assessment, 20*(2), 189–194.

Ferraro, V. A. (2013). *Immigrants and crime in the new destinations*. El Paso, TX: LFB Scholarly Publishing LLC.

Flanagan, D. P., & Ortiz, S. O. (2001). *Essentials of cross-battery assessment*. New York: John Wiley & Sons.

Flanagan, D. P., Ortiz, S. O., & Alfonso, V. C. (2017). Use of the cross-battery approach in the assessment of diverse individuals. In A. S. Kaufman (Ed.) & N. L. Kaufman (Series Ed.), *Essentials of cross-battery assessment second edition* (2nd ed., pp. 146–205). Hoboken, NJ: Wiley.

Foa, E. B., Johnson, K. M., Feeny, N. C., & Treadwell, K. R. (2001). The child PTSD symptom scale: A preliminary examination of its psychometric properties. *Journal of Clinical Child Psychology, 30*(3), 376–384. https://doi.org/10.1207/S15374424JCCP3003_9

Foa, E. B., Johnson, K. M., Feeny, N. C., & Treadwell, K. R. (2001). The child PTSD symptom scale: A preliminary examination of its psychometric properties. *Journal of Clinical Child Psychology, 30*(3), 376–384. https://doi.org/10.1207/S15374424JCCP3003_9

Foronda, C., Baptiste, D. L., Reinholdt, M. M., & Ousman, K. (2016). Cultural humility: A concept analysis. *Journal of Transcultural Nursing, 27*(3), 210–217.

Franklin, J. (2019). Coping with racial battle fatigue: differences and similarities for African American and Mexican American college students. *Race, Ethnicity, & Education, 22*(5), 589–609. doi:10.1080/13613324.2019.1579178

Galicia-Moreno, E. F., Francisco, R., Ulloa, R. E., Palacios-Cruz Sr, L., Ortiz, S. A., Palacio-Ortiz, J. D., Larraguibel, M., Abadi, A. F., Viola, L., & Felix, F. (2018). 3.12 Validity and reliability of the K-Sads present and lifetime version DSM-5 (K-SADS-PL-5) Spanish Version. *Journal of the American Academy of Child & Adolescent Psychiatry, 57*(10), S185. https://doi.org/10.1016/j.jaac.2018.09.170

García-Peltoniemi, R. E., & Azan Chiviano, A. (1993). MMPI-2: Inventario Multifásico de la Personalidad-2-Minnesota. *Minneapolis, MN: University of Minnesota Press, 239,* 15.

Garcini, L. M., Chen, M. A., Brown, R. L., Galvan, T., Saucedo, L., Berger Cardoso, J. A., & Fagundes, C. P. (2018). Kicks hurt less: Discrimination predicts distress beyond trauma among undocumented Mexican immigrants. *Psychology of Violence, 8*(6), 692. https://doi.org/10.1037/vio0000205

Garcini, L. M., Pham, T. T., Ambriz, A. M., Lill, S., & Tsevat, J. (2021a). COVID-19 diagnostic testing among underserved Latino communities: Barriers and facilitators. *Health & Social Care in the Community, 0,* 1–10. https://doi.org/10.1111/hsc.13621

Garrido, M., & Cabiya, J. J. (2013). Assessing Personality Using Self-Report Measures with Hispanic Clients. In L. T. Benuto (Ed.), *Guide to Psychological Assessment with Hispanics* (pp. 57–80). Springer, Boston, MA.

Geisinger, K. F., & Carlson, J. F. (1998). Training psychologists to assess members of a diverse society. In J. Sandoval, C. L. Frisby, K. F. Geisinger, J. D. Scheuneman, & J. R. Grenier (Eds.), *Test interpretation and diversity: Achieving equity in assessment* (pp. 375–386). Washington, DC: American Psychological Association. http://dx.doi.org/10.1037/10279-014

Geisinger, K. F. (2005). The testing industry, ethnic minorities, and those with disabilities. In R. Phelps (Ed.), *Defending standardized testing* (pp. 187–203). Mahwah, NJ: Erlbaum.

Geisinger, K. F. (2015). A brief review of Spanish-language adaptations of some English-language intelligence tests. In K.F. Geisinger (Ed.), *Psychological testing of Hispanics: Clinical, cultural, and intellectual issues* (2nd ed., pp. 135–152). Washington, DC: American Psychological Association.

Ghorpade, J., Hattrup, K., & Lackritz, J. R. (1999). The use of personality measures in cross-cultural research: A test of three personality scales across two countries. *Journal of Applied Psychology, 84*(5), 670–679. https://doi.org/10.1037/0021-9010.84.5.670

Gloria, A. M., Ruiz, E. L., & Castillo, E. M. (2004). Counseling and psychotherapy with Latino and Latina clients. In T. Smith (Ed.), *Practicing multiculturalism: Affirming diversity in counseling and psychology* (pp. 167–189). Boston: Allyn & Bacon.

González-Prendes, A. A., Hindo, C., & Pardo, Y. F. (2011). Cultural values integration in cognitive–behavioral therapy for a Latino with depression. *Clinical Case Studies, 10,* 376–394. http://dx.doi.org/10.1177/1534650111427075

Goodman, W. K., Price, L. H., Rasmussen, S. A., Mazure, C., Fleischmann, R. L., Hill, C. L., . . . Charney, D. S. (1989). The Yale Brown Obsessive Compulsive Scale. *Archives of General Psychiatry, 46,* 1006–1011.

Gould, J. B., Madan, A., Qin, C., & Chavez, G. (2003). Perinatal outcomes in two dissimilar immigrant populations in the United States: A dual epidemiologic paradox. *Pediatrics, 111*(6), 676–682. https://doi.org/10.1542/peds.111.6.e676

Greene, R. L. (1987). Ethnicity and MMPI performance: A review. *Journal of Consulting and Clinical Psychology, 55*(4), 497–512.

Gross, M., Buac, M., & Kaushanskaya, M. (2014). Conceptual scoring of receptive and expressive vocabulary measures in simultaneous and sequential bilingual children. *American Journal of Speech-Language Pathology, 23*(4), 574–586. https://doi.org/10.1044/2014_AJSLP-13-0026

Gross, D., Fogg, L., Young, M., Ridge, A., Cowell, J. M., Richardson, R., & Sivan, A. (2006). The equivalence of the Child Behavior Checklist/1 1/2-5 across parent race/ ethnicity, income level, and language. *Psychological Assessment, 18*(3), 313.

Guarnaccia, P. J., Martinez, I., & Acosta, H. (2005). Chapter 2. Mental health in the Hispanic immigrant community: An overview. *Journal of Immigrant & Refugee Services, 3*(1–2), 21–46.

Guarnaccia, P. J., Martinez, I., Ramirez, R., & Canino, G. (2005). Are ataques de nervios in Puerto Rican children associated with psychiatric disorder?. *Journal of the American Academy of Child & Adolescent Psychiatry, 44*(11), 1184–1192. https://doi.org/10.1097/01.chi.0000177059.34031.5d

Gudiño, O. G., & Rindlaub, L. A. (2014). Psychometric properties of the Child PTSD Symptom Scale in Latino children. *Journal of Traumatic Stress, 27*(1), 27–34.

Gutierrez, G. (2002). Ethnopsychological method and the psychological assessment of Mexican Americans. *Hispanic Journal of Behavioral Sciences, 24*(3), 259–277.

Gutierrez, P. M., Osman, A., Barrios, F. X., & Kopper, B. A. (2001). Development and initial validation of the Self-Harm Behavior Questionnaire. *Journal of Personality Assessment, 77*(3), 475–490.

Hale, S., Goodman-Delahunty, J., & Martschuk, N. (2019). Interpreter performance in police interviews: Differences between trained interpreters and untrained bilinguals. *The Interpreter and Translator Trainer, 13*(2), 107–131. doi:10.1080/1750399X.2018.1541649

Hall, G. C. N., Bansal, A., & Lopez, I. R. (1999). Ethnicity and psychopathology: A meta-analytic review of 31 years of comparative MMPI/MMPI-2 research. *Psychological Assessment, 11*(2), 186–197.

Hall, J. T., Menton, W. H., & Ben-Porath, Y. S. (2022). Examining the psychometric equivalency of MMPI-3 scale scores derived from the MMPI-3 and the MMPI-2-RF-EX. *Assessment, 29*(4), 842–853.

Hernandez-Cervantes, Q., & Gomez-Maqueo, E. L. (2006). Assessment of suicidal risk and associated stress in Mexican adolescent students. *Revista Mexicana De Psicologia, 23*(1), 45–52.

Handel, R. W., & Ben-Porath, Y. S. (2000). Multicultural assessment with the MMPI-2: Issues for research and practice. *Handbook of Cross-Cultural and Multicultural Personality Assessment,* 229–245.

Harris, C. (2004). Bilingual speakers in the lab: Psychophysiological measures of emotional reactivity. *Journal of Multilingual and Multicultural Development, 25*(2-3), 223–247. https://doi.org/10.1080/01434630408666530

Harris, C. L., Ayçíçeğí, A., & Gleason, J. B. (2003). Taboo words and reprimands elicit greater autonomic reactivity in a first language than in a second language. *Applied Psycholinguistics, 24*(4), 561–579. https://doi.org/10.1017/S0142716403000286

Heilemann, M. V., Kury, F. S., & Lee, K. A. (2005). Trauma and posttraumatic stress disorder symptoms among low income women of Mexican descent in the United States. *The Journal of Nervous and Mental Disease, 193*(10), 665–672.

Helms, J. E. (1992). Why is there no study of cultural equivalence in standardized cognitive ability testing? *American Psychologist, 47*(9), 1083–1101.

Hernández, B., Ramírez García, J. I., & Flynn, M. (2010). The role of familism in the relation between parent–child discord and psychological distress among emerging adults of Mexican descent. *Journal of Family Psychology, 24*(2), 105–114. https://doi.org/10.1037/a0019140

Hiskey, J. T., Córdova, A., Orcés, D., & Malone, M. F. (2016). Understanding the Central American refugee crisis: Why they are fleeing and how U.S. policies are failing to deter them. *American Immigration Council.* Retrieved from https://www.america

nimmigrationcouncil.org/sites/default/files/research/understanding_the_cent
ral_american_refugee_crisis.pdf

Hodes, M. (2000). Psychologically distressed refugee children in the United Kingdom.
Child Psychology and Psychiatry Review, 5(2), 57–68.

Homayounpour, G., & Movahedi, S. (2012). Transferential discourse in the language of
the (m) other. *Canadian Journal of Psychoanalysis, 20*(1), 114–143.

Homeland Security. (2002). *Homeland Security Act of 2002.* https://www.dhs.gov/homel
and-security-act-2002

Hook, J. N., Davis, D. E., Owens, J., Worthington, E. L., & Utsey, S. O. (2013). Cultural
humility: Measuring openness to culturally diverse clients. *Journal of Counseling
Psychology, 60*(3), 353–366.

Hooper, L. M., Stockton, P., Krupnick, J. L., & Green, B. L. (2011). Development, use,
and psychometric properties of the Trauma History Questionnaire. *Journal of Loss
and Trauma, 16*(3), 258–283.

Howe, M. L., Goodman, G. S., & Cicchetti, D. (Eds.). (2008). *Stress, trauma, and children's
memory development: Neurobiological, cognitive, clinical, and legal perspectives.*
Oxford University Press.

Hsu, C. T., Jacobs, A. M., & Conrad, M. (2015). Can Harry Potter still put a spell on us
in a second language? An fMRI study on reading emotion-laden literature in late
bilinguals. *Cortex, 63,* 282–295.

Hui, C. H., & Triandis, H. C. (1985). Measurement in cross-cultural psychology: A review and comparison of strategies. *Journal of Cross-Cultural Psychology, 16*(2), 131–
152. https://doi.org/10.1177/0022002185016002001

Hwang, W. C., & Ting, J. Y. (2008). Disaggregating the effects of acculturation and acculturative stress on the mental health of Asian Americans. *Cultural Diversity and
Ethnic Minority Psychology, 14*(2), 147.

Hwa-Froelich, D. A., & Westby, C. E. (2003). Considerations when working with
interpreters. *Communication Disorders Quarterly, 24*(2), 78–85. https://doi.org/
10.1177/15257401030240020401

Javier, R. A., Barroso, F., & Muñoz, M. A. (1993). Autobiographical memory in bilinguals.
Journal of Psycholinguistic Research, 22(3), 319–338. https://doi.org/10.1007/BF0
1068015

Jaycox, L. H., Stein, B. D., Kataoka, S. H., Wong, M., Fink, A., Escudero, P., & Zaragoza, C.
(2002). Violence exposure, posttraumatic stress disorder, and depressive symptoms
among recent immigrant schoolchildren. *Journal of The American Academy of Child
& Adolescent Psychiatry, 41*(9), 1104–1110.

Jenkins, S. R. (Ed.). (2008). *A handbook of scoring systems for thematic apperceptive
techniques.* New York: Erlbaum.

Karlsson, R. (2005). Ethnic matching between therapist and patient in psychotherapy: an
overview of findings, together with methodological and conceptual issues. *Cultural
Diversity and Ethnic Minority Psychology, 11*(2), 113. https://doi.org/10.1037/
1099-9809.11.2.113

Kassam-Adams, N., Marsac, M. L., Hildenbrand, A., & Winston, F. (2013). Posttraumatic
stress following pediatric injury: Update on diagnosis, risk factors, and intervention.
JAMA Pediatrics, 167(12), 1158–1165.

Kataoka, S. H., Langley, A., Stein, B., Jaycox, L., Zhang, L., Sanchez, N., & Wong, M.
(2009). Violence exposure and PTSD: The role of English language fluency in Latino
youth. *Journal of Child and Family Studies, 18*(3), 334–341.

Kataoka, S. H., Stein, B. D., Jaycox, L. H., Wong, M., Escudero, P., Tu, W., . . . Fink, A. (2003). A school-based mental health program for traumatized Latino immigrant children. *Journal of the American Academy of Child & Adolescent Psychiatry, 42*(3), 311–318.

Kaplan, M. S., & Marks, G. (1990). Adverse effects of acculturation: Psychological distress among Mexican American young adults. *Social Science & Medicine, 31*(12), 1313–1319.

Kaplan, R. M., & Saccuzzo, D. P. (2013). *Psychological testing: Principles, applications, and issues.* Boston: Wadsworth Cengage Learning.

Kennedy, T. M., & Ceballo, R. (2014). Who, what, when, and where? Toward a dimensional conceptualization of community violence exposure. *Review of General Psychology, 18*(2), 69–81. https://doi.org/10.1037/gpr0000005

Kermott, S. E. (2017). *Comparability of the English and Spanish Adaptation of the MMPI-2 Rf With US Bilingual Latinos* (Doctoral dissertation, Alliant International University).

Kinginger, C. (2004). Alice doesn't live here anymore: Foreign language learning and identity reconstruction. In A. Pavlenko & A. Blackledge (Eds.), *Negotiation of identities in multilingual contexts* (pp. 219–242). Bristol, Blue Ridge Summit: Multilingual Matters. https://doi.org/10.21832/9781853596483-010

Kisser, J. E., Wendell, C. R., Spencer, R. J., & Waldstein, S. R. (2012). Neuropsychological performance of native versus non-native English speakers. *Archives of Clinical Neuropsychology, 27*(7), 749–755. https://doi.org/10.1093/arclin/acs082

Khouri, R. (2010). *MMPI-2 RF vs. MMPI-2: Latinos with depression* (Doctoral dissertation, Alliant International University, California School of Professional Psychology, San Diego).

Knight, G. P., & Hill, N. E. (1998). Measurement equivalence in research involving minority adolescents. In V. C. McLoyd & L. Steinberg (Eds.), *Studying minority adolescents: Conceptual, methodological, and theoretical issues* (pp. 183–210). New York: Lawrence Erlbaum.

Knight, G. P., Tein, J., Prost, J. H., & Gonzales, N. A. (2002). Measurement equivalence and research on Latino children and families: The importance of culturally informed theory. In. J. M. Contreras, K. A. Kerns, & A. M. Neal-Barnett (Eds.), *Latino children and families in the United States: Current research and future directions.* Westport, CT: Greenwood.

Kondo, K. K., Rossi, J. S., Schwartz, S. J., Zamboanga, B. L., & Scalf, C. D. (2016). Acculturation and cigarette smoking in Hispanic women: A meta-analysis. *Journal of Ethnicity in Substance Abuse, 15*(1), 46–72.

Kouyoumdjian, H., Zamboanga, B. L., & Hansen, D. J. (2003). Barriers to community mental health services for Latinos: Treatment considerations. *Clinical Psychology: Science and Practice, 10*(4), 394–422. https://doi.org/10.1093/clipsy.bpg041

Kranzler, J. H., Flores, C. G., & Coady, M. (2010). Examination of the cross-battery approach for the cognitive assessment of children and youth from diverse linguistic and cultural backgrounds. *School Psychology Review, 39*(3), 431–446.

Labouvie, E., & Ruetsch, C. (1995). Testing for equivalence of measurement scales: Simple structure and metric invariance reconsidered. *Multivariate Behavioral Research, 30*(1), 63–76. https://doi.org/10.1207/s15327906mbr3001_4

La Roche, M. J. (2013). *Cultural psychotherapy: Theory, methods, and practice*. Thousand Oaks, CA: Sage Publications.

Larry P. v. Riles, 343 F. Supp. 1306 (N.D. Cal. 1972), aff'd 502 F. 2d 963 (9th Cir. 1974); 495 F. Supp. 926 (N.D. Cal. 1979), aff'd 793 F. 2d 969 (9th Cir. 1984).

Lewis-Fernandez, R., Horvitz-Lenon, M., Blanco, C., Guarnaccia, P., Cao, Z., & Alegria, M. (2009). Significance of endorsement of psychotic symptoms by U.S. Latinos. *Journal of Nervous and Mental Disease, 197*, 337–347.

Livingston G. (2009, September 25). Hispanics, Health Insurance and Health Care Access. Pew Hispanic Center. https://www.pewresearch.org/hispanic/2009/09/25/hispanics-health-insurance-and-health-care-access/

Locke, C. J., Southwick, K., McCloskey, L. A., & Fernández-Esquer, M. E. (1996). The psychological and medical sequelae of war in Central American refugee mothers and children. *Archives of pediatrics & adolescent medicine, 150*(8), 822–828. https://doi.org/10.1001/archpedi.1996.02170330048008

Lohman, D. F., Korb, K., Lakin, J. (2008). Identifying academically gifted English language learners using nonverbal tests: A comparison of the Raven, NNAT, and CogAT. *Gifted Child Quarterly, 52*, 275–296.

López, E. J., Ehly, S., & García-Vásquez, E. (2002). Acculturation, social support and academic achievement of Mexican and Mexican American high school students: An exploratory study. *Psychology in the Schools, 39*, 245–257. http://dx.doi.org/10.1002/pits.10009

Lopez, S., & Romero, A. (1988). Assessing the intellectual functioning of Spanish-speaking adults: Comparison of the EIWA and the WAIS. Professional Psychology: *Research and Practice, 19*(3), 263–270.

Lui, P. P. (2015). Intergenerational cultural conflict, mental health, and educational outcomes among Asian and Latino/a Americans: Qualitative and meta-analytic review. *Psychological Bulletin, 141*(2), 404–446. https://doi.org/10.1037/a0038449

Lucio, E., Ampudia, A., Durán, C., León, I., & Butcher, J. N. (2001). Comparison of the Mexican and American norms of the MMPI2. *Journal of Clinical Psychology, 57*(12), 1459–1468.

Lucio, G. M. E., Palacios, H., Durán, C., & Butcher, J. N. (1999). MMPI-2 with mexican psychiatric inpatients: Basic and content scales. *Journal of Clinical Psychology, 55*(12), 1541–1552.

Lucio, G. M. E., Reyes-Lagunes, I., & Scott, R. L. (1994). MMPI-2 for Mexico: Translation and adaptation. *Journal of Personality Assessment, 63*(1), 105–116.

Lucio, E., & Reyes, I. (1994). La nueva versión del Inventario Multifásico de la Personalidad de Minnesota MMPI-2 para estudiantes universitarios mexicanos. *Revista Mexicana de Psicología, 11*(1), 45–54.

Lund, D., & Lee, L. (2015). Fostering cultural humility among pre-service teachers: Connecting with children and youth of immigrant families through service-learning. *Canadian Journal of Education / Revue Canadienne De L'éducation, 38*(2), 1–30. https://doi.org/10.2307/canajeducrevucan.38.2.10

MacDonald, J., & Saunders, J. (2012). Are immigrant youth less violent? Specifying the reasons and mechanisms. *The Annals of the American Academy of Political and Social Science, 641*(1), 125–147. https://doi.org/10.1177/0002716211432279

Mahurin, R. K., Espino, D., & Holifield, E. B. (1992). Mental status testing in elderly Hispanic population: Special concerns. *Psychopharmacology Bulletin, 28*, 391–399.

Maldonado, C. Y., & Geisinger, K. F. (2005). Conversion of the Wechsler Adult Intelligence Scale into Spanish: An early test adaption effort of considerable consequence. In R. K. Hambleton, P. F. Merenda, C. D. Spielberg (Eds.), *Adapting Educational and psychological tests for cross cultural assessment* (pp 213–234). Hillsdale: Erlbaum.

Maramba, G. G., & Nagayama Hall, G. C. (2002). Meta-analyses of ethnic match as a predictor of dropout, utilization, and level of functioning. *Cultural Diversity and Ethnic Minority Psychology*, *8*(3), 290. https://doi.org/10.1037/1099-9809.8.3.290

Marin, G., Sabogal, F., Marin, B. V., Otero-Sabogal, R., & Perez-Stable, E. J. (1987). Development of a short acculturation scale for Hispanics. *Hispanic Journal of Behavioral Sciences*, *9*(2), 183–205.

Marshall, K., & Venta, A. (2021). Psychometric evaluation of the caregiver version of the Child PTSD Symptom Scale in a recently immigrated, Spanish speaking population. *Psychiatry Research*, *301*, 113954.

Martinez, C. (2013). Conducting the cross-cultural clinical interview. In *Handbook of Multicultural Mental Health* (pp. 191–204). Academic Press.

Matsumoto, D., & Kupperbusch, C. (2001). Idiocentric and allocentric differences in emotional expression, experience, and the coherence between expression and experience. *Asian Journal of Social Psychology*, *4*(2), 113–131. https://doi.org/10.1111/j.1467-839X.2001.00080.x

Maulik, P. K., Daniels, A. M., McBain, R., & Morris, J. M. (2014). Global mental health resources. In V. Patel, H. Minas, A. Cohen & M. J. Prince (Eds.), *Global mental health: Principles and practice* (pp. 167–192). Oxford.

Maqueo, E. L. G., & Arenas-Landgrave, P. (2013). Special Considerations When Assessing the Hispanic Adolescent: Examining Suicide Risk. In *Guide to Psychological Assessment with Hispanics* (pp. 129–139). Springer: Boston, MA.

Mbroh, H., Najjab, A., Knap, S., & Gottlieb, M. C. (2019). Prejudiced patients: Ethical considerations for addressing patient's prejudicial comments in psychotherapy. *Professional Psychology: Research and Practice*, *51*(3), 284–290.

McCloskey, D. M., Hess, R. S., & D'Amato, R. C. (2003). Evaluating the utility of the Spanish version of the Behavior Assessment System for Children-Parent report system. *Journal of Psychoeducational Assessment*, *21*(4), 325–337.

McGrew, K. S., & Flanagan, D. P. (1998). *The intelligence test desk reference (ITDR): Gf-Gc cross-battery assessment*. Boston: Allyn & Bacon.

McLaughlin, K. A., Hilt, L. M., & Nolen-Hoeksema, S. (2007). Racial/ethnic differences in internalizing and externalizing symptoms in adolescents. *Journal of Abnormal Child Psychology*, *35*(5), 801–816. https://doi.org/10.1007/s10802-007-9128-1

McNamara, T. F. (1997). 'Interaction' in second language performance assessment: Whose performance? *Applied Linguistics*, *18*(4), 446–466. https://doi.org/10.1093/applin/18.4.446

Melendez, F. (1994). The Spanish version of the WAIS: Some ethical considerations. *The Clinical Neuropsychologist*, *8*(4), 388–393.

Mercado, A., Antuna, C, Bailey, C., Garcini, L., Hass, G. A., Henderson, C., Koslofsky, S., Morales, F., & Venta, A. (July, 2022). Professional Guidelines for Psychological Evaluations in Immigration Proceedings. *Journal of Latinx Psychology*. http://dx.doi.org/10.1037/lat0000209

Mercado, A., & Hinojosa, Y. (2017). Culturally adapted dialectical behavior therapy in an underserved community mental health setting: A Latina adult case study. *Practice Innovations*, *2*(2), 80–93. https://doi.org/10.1037/pri0000045

Mercado, A., Venta, A., Henderson, C., & Pimentel, N. (2019). Trauma and cultural values in the health of recently immigrated families. *Journal of Health Psychology*, *26*(5), 728–740. https://doi.org/10.1177/1359105319842935

Mercado, A., Venta, A., & Irizarry, R. (2019). Best practice and research perspectives with immigrant groups. In M. Zangeneh & A. Al-Krenawi (Eds.), *Culture, diversity, and mental health-enhancing clinical practice* (pp. 83–106). Cham: Springer.

Meyer, E. L. (2013). *Diagnostic accuracy of the Culture-Language Interpretive Matrix with the WJ-III-NU: A comparison of Spanish-speaking English language learners and monolingual English-speaking students.* [Doctoral dissertation, The Pennsylvania State University].

Meyer, G. J., Finn, S. E., Eyde, L. D., Kay, G. G., Moreland, K. L., Dies, R. R., . . . Reed, G. M. (2001). Psychological testing and psychological assessment: A review of evidence and issues. *American psychologist*, *56*(2), 128.

Meyer, G. J., Shaffer, T. W., Erdberg, P., & Horn, S. L. (2015). Addressing issues in the development and use of the Composite International Reference Values as Rorschach norms for adults. *Journal of Personality Assessment*, *97*(4), 330–347.

Mezzich, J. E., Caracci, G., Fabrega, H., & Kirmayer, L. J. (2009). Cultural formulation guidelines. *Transcultural Psychiatry*, *46*(3), 383–405.

Miller, L. A., & Loveler, R. L. (2020). *Foundations of psychological testing: A practical approach.* Los Angeles: Sage.

Millett, L. S. (2016). The healthy immigrant paradox and child maltreatment: A systematic review. *Journal of Immigrant and Minority Health*, *18*(5), 1199–1215. https://doi.org/10.1007/s10903-016-0373-7

Mills, S., Xiao, A. X., Wolitzky-Taylor, K., Lim, R., & Lu, F. G. (2017). Training on the DSM5 Cultural Formulation Interview improves cultural competence in general psychiatry residents: A pilot study. *Transcultural Psychiatry*, *54*(2), 179–191.

Millsap, R. E., & Yun-Tein, J. (2004). Assessing factorial invariance in ordered-categorical measures. *Multivariate Behavioral Research*, *39*(3), 479–515. https://doi.org/10.1207/S15327906MBR3903_4

Miranda, J., Bernal, G., Lau, A., Kohn, L., Hwang, W. C., & LaFromboise, T. (2005). State of the science on psychosocial interventions for ethnic minorities. *Annual Review of Clinical Psychology*, *1*, 113–142. https://doi.org/10.1146/annurev.clinpsy.1.102803.143822

Miville, M. L., & Constantine, M. G. (2006). Sociocultural predictors of psychological help-seeking attitudes and behavior among Mexican American college students. *Cultural Diversity and Ethnic Minority Psychology*, *12*(3), 420.

Morey, L. C. (1991). *Personality assessment inventory.* Odessa, FL: Psychological Assessment Resources.

Morey, L. C. (2004). The Personality Assessment Inventory (PAI). In M. E. Maruish (Ed.), *The use of psychological testing for treatment planning and outcomes assessment: Instruments for adults* (pp. 509–551). Lawrence Erlbaum.

Mollica, R. F., Caspi-Yavin, Y., Bollini, P., Truong, T., Tor, S., & Lavelle, J. (1992). The Harvard Trauma Questionnaire: Validating a cross-cultural instrument for measuring torture, trauma, and posttraumatic stress disorder in Indochinese refugees. *Journal of Nervous and Mental Disease*, *180*(2), 111–116.

Mosher, D. K., Hook, J. N., Captari, L. E., Davis, D. E., DeBlaere, C., & Owen, J. (2017). Cultural humility: A therapeutic framework for engaging diverse clients. *Practice Innovations*, *2*(4), 221. https://doi.org/10.1037/pri0000055

Muñoz-Sandoval, A. F., Woodcock, R. W., McGrew, K. S., Mather, N. (2005). *Bateria III Woodcock- Muñoz*. Rolling Meadows: Riverside.

Muñoz, C., & Venta, A. (2019). Referring unaccompanied minors to psychiatric residential treatment: When is it worth the disruption to adaptation and shelter integration? *Residential Treatment for Children & Youth, 36*(2), 137–156. https://doi.org/10.1080/0886571X.2018.1524736

Nadal, K. L., Griffin, K. E., Wong, Y., Hamit, S., & Rasmus, M. (2014). The impact of racial microaggressions on mental health: Counseling implications for clients of color. *Journal of Counseling & Development, 92*(1), 57–66. https://doi.org/10.1002/j.1556-6676.2014.00130.x

National Association of Social Workers. (2021). Code of ethics of the National Association of Social Workers. Retrieved from https://www.socialworkers.org/About/Ethics/Code-of-Ethics/Code-of-Ethics-English

Nielsen, J. D. J., Wall, W., & Tucker, C. M. (2016). Testing of a model with Latino patients that explains the links among patient-perceived provider cultural sensitivity, language preference, and patient treatment adherence. *Journal of Racial and Ethnic Health Disparities, 3*(1), 63–73. https://doi.org/10.1007/s40615-015-0114-y

Nijad, F. (2003). A day in the life of an interpreting service. In R. Tribe & H. Raval (Eds.), *Undertaking mental health work using interpreters* (pp. 77–91). Routledge.

Noe-Bustamante, L. (2019). *Key factors about U.S. Hispanics and their diverse heritage*. Pew Research Center. https://www.pewresearch.org/fact-tank/2019/09/16/key-facts-about-u-s-hispanics/

Norcross, J. C., VandenBos, G. R., & Freedheim, D. K. (Eds.). (2016). *APA handbook of clinical psychology*. American Psychological Association.

Ochoa, S. H., & Ortiz, S. O. (2005). Cognitive assessment of culturally and linguistically diverse individuals: An integrative approach. In R. L. Rhodes, S. H Ochoa, & S. O. Ortiz (Eds.), *Assessing culturally and linguistically diverse individuals: A practical guide* (pp. 168–201). New York: Guilford Press.

Office of Refugee Resettlement (ORR). (2015). *Annual report to Congress*. Retrieved from https://www.acf.hhs.gov/sites/default/files/documents/orr/arc_15_final_508.pdf

Olvera, P., & Gomez-Cerrillo, L. (2011). A bilingual (English & Spanish) psychoeducational assessment MODEL grounded in Cattell-Horn Carroll (CHC) theory: A cross battery approach. *Contemporary School Psychology, 15*, 117–127. https://doi.org/10.1007/BF03340968

Ortiz, S. O., Ochoa, S. H., & Dynda, A. M. (2012). Testing with culturally and linguistically diverse populations: Moving beyond the verbal-performance dichotomy into evidence-based practice. In D. P. Flanagan & P. L. Harrison (Eds.), *contemporary intellectual assessment: Theories, tests, and issues* (3rd ed., pp. 526–552). New York: Guilford Press.

Osório, F. L., Loureiro, S. R., Hallak, J. E. C., Machado-de-Sousa, J. P., Ushirohira, J. M., Baes, C. V., . . . Crippa, J. A. S. (2019). Clinical validity and inter-rater and test-retest reliability of the Structured Clinical Interview for the DSM5-Clinical Version (SCID-5-CV). *Psychiatry and Clinical Neurosciences, 73*, 754–760.

Othmer, E., & Othmer, S. C. (2002). *The clinical interview using the DSMIV-TR. Volume 1: Fundamentals*. Washington, DC: American Psychiatric.

Padilla, R., Gomez, V., Biggerstaff, S., & Mehler, P. (2001). Use of Curanderismo in a public health care system. *Archives of Internal Medicine, 161*, 1336–1340.

Paniagua, F. A. (2005). *Assessing and treating culturally diverse clients: A practical guide* (3rd ed.). Thousand Oaks: Sage.

Paralikar, V.P, Deshmukh, A., & Weiss, M. G. (2019). Qualitative analysis of the Cultural Formulation Interview: Findings and implications for revising the outline for cultural formulation. *Transcultural Psychiatry, 0*(0), 1–29.

Parra-Cardona, J. R., López-Zerón, G., Domenech Rodríguez, M. M., Escobar-Chew, A. R., Whitehead, M. R., Sullivan, C. M., & Bernal, G. (2016). A balancing act: Integrating evidence-based knowledge and cultural relevance in a program of prevention parenting research with Latino/a immigrants. *Family Process, 55*(2), 321–337. https://doi.org/10.1111/famp.12190

Passel, J. S., Cohn, D. V., & Gonzalez-Barrera, A. (2013). Population decline of unauthorized immigrants stalls, may have reversed. Pew Research Center. https://www.pewresearch.org/hispanic/2013/09/23/population-decline-of-unauthorized-immigrants-stalls-may-have-reversed/

Patel, S. G., Clarke, A. V., Eltareb, F., Macciomei, E. E., & Wickham, R. E. (2016). Newcomer immigrant adolescents: A mixed-methods examination of family stressors and school outcomes. *School Psychology Quarterly, 31*(2), 163.

Pavlenko, A. (2006). Bilingual selves. In A. Pavlenko (Ed.), *Bilingual minds: Emotional experience, expression, and representation* (pp. 1–33). Bristol, Blue Ridge Summit: Multilingual Matters. https://doi.org/10.21832/9781853598746-003

Perreira, K. M., & Ornelas, I. (2013). Painful passages: Traumatic experiences and post-traumatic stress among immigrant Latino adolescents and their primary caregivers. *The International migration review, 47*(4), 10.1111/imre.12050. https://doi.org/10.1111/imre.12050

Pieterse, A. L., & Miller, M. J. (2009). Current considerations in the assessment of adults: A review and extension of culturally inclusive models. In J. Ponterotto, L. A. Suzuki, C. Alexander, & J. M. Cases (Eds.), *Handbook of multicultural counseling* (3rd ed., pp. 649–666). Thousand Oaks: Sage.

Pina, A. A., Gonzales, N. A., Holly, L. E., Zerr, A. A., & Wynne, H. (2013). Toward evidence-based clinical assessment of ethnic minority youth. In B. D. McLeod, A. Jensen-Doss, & T. H. Ollendick (Eds.), *Diagnostic and behavioral assessment in children and adolescents: A clinical guide* (pp. 348–376). New York: Guilford Press.

Pina, A. A., Little, M., Knight, G. P., & Silverman, W. K. (2009). Cross-ethnic measurement equivalence of the RCMAS in Latino and White youth with anxiety disorders. *Journal of Personality Assessment, 91*(1), 58–61. https://doi.org/10.1080/00223890802484183

Ponton, M. O., Gonzalez, J. J., Hernandez, I., Herrera, L., & Higareda, I. (2000). Factor analysis of the Neuropsychological Screening Battery for Hispanics (NeSBHIS). *Applied Neuropsychology, 7*(1), 32–39.

Potochnick, S. R., & Perreira, K. M. (2010). Depression and anxiety among first-generation immigrant Latino youth: Key correlates and implications for future research. *The Journal of Nervous and Mental Disease, 198*(7), 470–477. https://doi.org/10.1097/NMD.0b013e3181e4ce24

Puente, A. E., Ojeda, C., Zink, D., & Portillo Reyes, V. (2015). Neuropsychological testing of Spanish speakers. In K. F. Geisinger (Ed.), *Psychological testing of Hispanics: Clinical, cultural, and intellectual issues* (pp. 135–152). American Psychological Association. https://doi.org/10.1037/14668-008

Puente, A., & Perez-Garcia, M. (2000). Neuropsychological assessment of ethnic minorities. In I. Cuellar & F. A. Paniagua (Eds.), *Handbook of multicultural mental health: Assessment and treatment of diverse populations* (pp. 225–241). San Diego: Elsevier.

Pynoos, R. S., Frederick, C., Nader, K., Arroyo, W., Steinberg, A., Eth, S., . . . Fairbanks, L. (1987). Life threat and posttraumatic stress in school-age children. *Archives of General Psychiatry, 44*(12), 1057–1063.

Ramirez, J. D. (1991). Final report: Longitudinal study of structured English immersion strategy. *Bilingual Research Journal, 16*(1 & 2), 1–62.

Ramirez-Stege, A. M., Yarris, K. E. (2017). Culture in la clinica: Evaluating the utility of the Cultural Formulation Interview (CFI) in a Mexican outpatient setting. *Transcultural Psychiatry, 54*(4), 466–487.

Ranson, M. B., Nichols, D. S., Rouse, S. V., & Harrington, J. L. (2009). Changing or replacing an established psychological assessment standard: Issues, goals, and problems with special reference to recent developments in the MMPI-2. In J. N. Butcher (Ed.), *Oxford handbook of personality assessment* (pp. 112–139). Oxford University Press.

Rasmussen, A., Verkuilen, J., Ho, E., & Fan, Y. (2015). Posttraumatic stress disorder among refugees: Measurement invariance of Harvard Trauma Questionnaire scores across global regions and response patterns. *Psychological Assessment, 27*(4), 1160.

Renteria, L. (2010). Current practices survey on the neuropsychological assessment of Hispanics in the US. In First meeting of the Hispanic Neuropsychological Society, Acapulco, Mexico.

Raykov, T. (2004). Behavioral scale reliability and measurement invariance evaluation using latent variable modeling. *Behavior Therapy, 35*(2), 299–331. https://doi.org/10.1016/S0005-7894(04)80041-8

Reynolds, C. R., & Kamphaus, R. W. (2004). *Behavior assessment system for children* (2nd ed.). Circle Pines, MN: American Guidance Service.

Reed, R. V., Fazel, M., Jones, L., Panter-Brick, C., & Stein, A. (2012). Mental health of displaced and refugee children resettled in low-income and middle-income countries: Risk and protective factors. *Lancet (London, England), 379*(9812), 250–265. https://doi.org/10.1016/S0140-6736(11)60050-0

Reynaga-Abiko, G. (2005). *Towards a culturally relevant assessment of psychopathology with Mexicans/Mexican Americans* (Unpublished doctoral dissertation). Pepperdine University, Malibu, CA.

Reynaga-Abiko, G., Alamilla, S. G., Consoli, A. J., & Aros, J. (2016). Psychological testing and assessment of Latina/os. In F. T. L. Leong & Y. S. Park (Eds.), *Testing and Assessment with Persons & Communities of Color* (pp. 20–30). Washington, DC: American Psychological Association. https://www.apa.org/pi/oema

Reynolds, W. M. (1987). *Suicidal ideation questionnaire (SIQ)*. Odessa, FL: Psychological Assessment Resources.

Reynolds, W. (1991). *ASIQ, adult suicidal ideation questionnaire: professional manual.* Psychological Assessment Resources, Incorporated.

Rhodes, R. L., Ochoa, S. H., & Ortiz, S. O. (2005). *Assessing culturally and linguistically diverse students: A practical guide.* New York: Guilford Press.

Rivera, L. M. (2008). Acculturation and multicultural assessment: Issues, trends, and practice. In L. A. Suzuki & J. G. Ponterotto (Eds.), *Handbook of multicultural assessment* (3rd ed., pp. 73–91). San Francisco: Jossey-Bass.

Rissetti, F. J., Himmel, E., & Gonzalez-Moreno, J. A. (1996). Use of the MMPI-2 in Chile: Translation and adaptation. *International Adaptations of the MMPI-2: Research and Clinical Applications*, 221–251.

Rogers, R., Flores, J., Ustad, K., & Sewell, K. W. (1995). Initial validation of the personality assessment inventory—Spanish version with clients from Mexican American communities. *Journal of Personality Assessment, 64*(2), 340–348.

Rosenblum, M. R., & Ball, I. (2016). *Trends in unaccompanied child and family migration from Central America.* Washington, DC: Migration Policy Institute.

Ruiz, J. M., Hamann, H. A., Mehl, M. R., & O'Connor, M.-F. (2016). The Hispanic health paradox: From epidemiological phenomenon to contribution opportunities for psychological science. *Group Processes & Intergroup Relations, 19*(4), 462–476. https://doi.org/10.1177/1368430216638540

Ryder, A. G., Alden, L. E., & Paulhus, D. L. (2000). Is acculturation unidimensional or bidimensional? A head-to-head comparison in the prediction of personality, self-identity and adjustment. *Journal of Personality and Social Psychology, 79*(1), 49–65.

Sabogal, F., Marin, G., Otero-Sabogal, R., Marin, B. V., & Perez-Stable, E. J. (1987). Hispanic familism and acculturation: What changes and what doesn't? *Hispanic Journal of Behavioral Sciences, 9*(4), 397–412.

Saldana, D. (1992). Coping with stress: A refugee's story. *Women and Therapy, 13*, 21–34.

Sam, D. L., & Berry, J. W. (2010). Acculturation: When individuals and groups of different cultural backgrounds meet. *Perspectives on Psychological Science, 5*(4), 472–481. https://doi.org/10.1177/1745691610373075

SAMHSA. (2020). Double Jeopardy: COVID-19 and Behavioral Health Disparities for Black and Latino Communities in the U.S. https://www.samhsa.gov/sites/default/files/covid19-behavioral-health-disparities-black-latino-communities.pdf

Sanchez, G. I. (1932). Group differences and Spanish speaking children: A critical review. *Journal of Applied Psychology, 16*(5), 549–558.

Sanchez, G. I. (1934). Bilingualism and mental health measures. *Journal of Applied Psychology, 18*, 765.

Sanchez-Escobedo, P., Hollingworth, L., & Fina, A. D. (2011). Cross cultural, comparative study of the American, Spanish and Mexican versions of the WISCIV. *TESOL Quarterly, 45*(4), 781–792.

Satcher, D. (2001). *Mental health: Culture, race, and ethnicity—A supplement to mental health: A report of the surgeon general.* US Department of Health and Human Services. Retrieved from http://hdl.handle.net/1903/22834

Schraufnagel, T. J., Wagner, A. W., Miranda, J., & Roy-Byrne, P. P. (2006). Treating minority patients with depression and anxiety: What does the evidence tell us? *General Hospital Psychiatry, 28*(1), 27–36.

Schrank, F. A., McGrew, K. S., Ruef, M. L., & Alvarado, C. G. (2005). *Batería III Woodcock-Muñoz.* Rolling Meadows: Riverside Publishing.

Schrank, F. A., McGrew, K. S., Ruef, M. L., Alvarado, C. G., Muñoz-Sandoval, A. F., & Woodcock, R. W. (2005). *Overview and technical supplement (Batería III Woodcock-Muñoz Assessment Service Bulletin No. 1).* Itasca, IL: Riverside Publishing.

Schuessler, J. B., Wilder, B., & Byrd, L. W. (2012). Reflecting journaling and development of cultural humility in students. *Nursing Education Perspectives, 33*(2), 96–99.

Schwartz, S. J., Unger, J. B., Zamboanga, B. L., & Szapocznik, J. (2010). Rethinking the concept of acculturation: Implications for theory and research. *American Psychologist, 65*(4), 237–251. https://doi.org/10.1037/a0019330

Searight, H. R., & Armock, J. A. (2013). Foreign language interpreters in mental health: A literature review and research agenda. *North American Journal of Psychology, 15*(1), 17–38.

Shaffer, D., Scott, M., Wilcox, H., Maslow, C., Hicks, R., Lucas, C. P., . . . Greenwald, S. (2004). The Columbia SuicideScreen: Validity and reliability of a screen for youth suicide and depression. *Journal of the American Academy of Child & Adolescent Psychiatry, 43*(1), 71–79.

Smokowski, P. R., & Bacallao, M. L. (2006). Acculturation and aggression in Latino adolescents: A structural model focusing on cultural risk factors and assets. *Journal of Abnormal Child Psychology, 34*(5), 657–671.

Sotelo-Dynega, M., Ortiz, S. O., Flanagan, D. P., & Chaplin, W. F. (2013), English language proficiency and test performance: An evaluation of bilingual students with the Woodcock-Johnson III Tests of Cognitive Abilities. *Psychology in the Schools, 50*, 781–797. https://doi.org/10.1002/pits.21706

Steinberg, A. M., Brymer, M. J., Decker, K. B., & Pynoos, R. S. (2004). The University of California at Los Angeles post-traumatic stress disorder reaction index. *Current Psychiatry Reports, 6*(2), 96–100.

Stinchcomb, D., & Hershberg, E. (2014). *Unaccompanied migrant children from Central America: Context, causes, and responses.* Washington, DC: American University Center for Latin American & Latino Studies.

Styck, K. M., & Watkins, M. W. (2014). Discriminant validity of the WISC-IV Culture-Language Interpretive Matrix. *Contemporary School Psychology, 18*(3), 168–177. https://doi.org/10.1007/s40688-014-0021-y

Suárez-Orozco, C., Rhodes, J., & Milburn, M. (2009). Unraveling the immigrant paradox: Academic engagement and disengagement among recently arrived immigrant youth. *Youth & Society, 41*(2), 151–185. https://doi.org/10.1177/0044118X09333647

Suárez-Orozco, C. (2001). Afterword: Understanding and serving the children of immigrants. *Harvard Educational Review, 71*(3), 579–590.

Sue, D. W. (2010). *Microaggressions in everyday life: Race, gender, and sexual orientation.* Hoboken: Wiley.

Sue, S. (1988). Psychotherapeutic services for ethnic minorities: Two decades of research findings. *American Psychologist, 43*(4), 301. https://doi.org/10.1037/0003-066X.43.4.301

Suen, H. K., & Greenspan, S. (2009). Serious problems with the Mexican norms for the WAIS-III when assessing for mental retardation in capital cases. *Applied Neuropsychology, 16*(3), 214–222. http://dx.doi.org/10.1080/09084280903098786

Tafur, M., Crowe, T., & Torres, E. (2009). A review of curanderismo and healing practices among Mexicans and Mexican Americans. *Occupational Therapy International, 16*(1), 82–88. doi:10.1002/oti.265

Teruya, S. A., & Bazargan-Hejazi, S. (2013). The immigrant and Hispanic paradoxes: A systematic review of their predictions and effects. *Hispanic Journal of Behavioral Sciences, 35*(4), 486–509. https://doi.org/10.1177/0739986313499004

The Covidtracking Project (2020). Retried from https://covidtracking.com/

Tormala, T. T., Patel, S. G., Soukup, E. E., & Clarke, A. V. (2018). Developing measurable cultural competence and cultural humility: An application of the cultural formulation. *Training and Education in Professional Psychology, 12*(1), 54. https://doi.org/10.1037/tep0000183

Tribe, R., & Raval, H. (2003). *Undertaking mental health work using interpreters.* Routledge.

Turner, E. A., Cheng, H.-L., Llamas, J. D., Tran, A. G. T. T., Hill, K. X., Fretts, J. M., & Mercado, A. (2016). Factors impacting the current trends in the use of outpatient psychiatric treatment among diverse ethnic groups. *Current Psychiatry Reviews, 12*(2), 199–220. https://doi.org/10.2174/1573400512666160216234524

Turner, R. J., Lloyd, D. A., & Taylor, J. (2006). Stress burden, drug dependence and the nativity paradox among US Hispanics. *Drug and Alcohol Dependence, 83*(1), 79–89.

UN General Assembly. (1951). *Convention Relating to the Status of Refugees.* United Nations. https://www.refworld.org/docid/3be01b964.html

UN High Commissioner for Refugees (UNHCR). (2012). *Report of the United Nations High Commissioner for Refugees – 2012.* https://www.refworld.org/docid/509a60 4e2.html

UN High Commissioner for Refugees (UNHCR). (2017). *Global Trends: Forced Displacement in 2017.* https://www.refworld.org/docid/5b2d1a867.html

US Census Bureau. (2011). Selected characteristics of the native and foreign-born population by period of entry into the United States. Retrieved from https://data.census. gov/cedsci/table?q=foreign%20born&tid=ACSST1Y2011.S0502

US Customs and Border Protection. (2021). CBP enforcement statistics fiscal year 2021. Retrieved from https://www.cbp.gov/newsroom/stats/cbp-enforcement-statistics

Vandenberg, R. J., & Lance, C. E. (2000). A review and synthesis of the measurement invariance literature: Suggestions, practices, and recommendations for organizational research. *Organizational Research Methods, 3*(1), 4–70. https://doi.org/10.1177/ 109442810031002

Van Deth, L. M. (2013). *Validity of the KABC-II Culture-Language Interpretive Matrix: A comparison of native English speakers and Spanish-speaking English language learners.* [Doctoral dissertation/The Pennsylvania State University]. ProQuest.

Van de Vijver, F. J. R., & Leung, K. (2011). Equivalence and bias: A review of concepts, models, and data analytic procedures. In D. Matsumoto & F. J. R. van de Vijver (Eds.), *Cross-cultural research methods in psychology* (pp. 17–45). Cambridge: Cambridge University Press.

Vasquez-Guzman, C. E., Hess, J. M., Casas, N., Medina, D., Galvis, M., Torres, D. A., . . . Goodkind, J. R. (2020). Latinx/@ immigrant inclusion trajectories: Individual agency, structural constraints, and the role of community-based organizations in immigrant mobilities. *American Journal of Orthopsychiatry, 90*(6), 772.

Velasquez, R. J., Gonzales, M., Butcher, J. N., Castillo-Canez, I., Apodaca, J. X., & Chavira, D. (1997). Use of the MMPI-2 with Chicanos: Strategies for counselors. *Journal of Multicultural Counseling and Development, 25*(2), 107–120.

Velasquez, R. J., Chavira, D. A., Karle, H. R., Callahan, W. J., Garcia, J. A., & Castellanos, J. (2000). Assessing bilingual and monolingual Latino students with translations of the MMPI-2: Initial data. *Cultural Diversity and Ethnic Minority Psychology, 6*(1), 65–72.

Venta A. (2019). The real emergency at our southern border is mental health. *Journal of the American Academy of Child and Adolescent Psychiatry, 58*(12), 1217–1218. https://doi.org/10.1016/j.jaac.2019.05.029

Venta, A., Bick, J., & Bechelli, J. (2021). COVID-19 threatens maternal mental health and infant development: possible paths from stress and isolation to adverse outcomes and a call for research and practice. *Child Psychiatry & Human Development*, *52*(2), 200–204. https://doi.org/10.1007/s10578-021-01140-7

Venta, A., Muñoz, C., & Bailey, C. (2017). What language does your internal working model of attachment speak? *Journal of Cross-Cultural Psychology*, *48*(6), 813–834. https://doi.org/10.1177/0022022117704053

Venta, A. C., & Mercado, A. (2019). Trauma screening in recently immigrated youth: Data from two Spanish-speaking samples. *Journal of Child and Family Studies*, *28*(1), 84–90. https://doi.org/10.1007/s10826-018-1252-8

Venta, A. C., & Mercado, A. (2019). Trauma screening in recently immigrated youth: Data from two Spanish-speaking samples. *Journal of Child and Family Studies*, *28*(1), 84–90. https://doi.org/10.1007/s10826-018-1252-8

Venta, A. (2020). Attachment facilitates acculturative learning and adversity moderates: Validating the theory of epistemic trust in a natural experiment. *Child Psychiatry & Human Development*, *51*, 471–477. https://doi.org/10.1007/s10 578-020-00958-x

Villatoro, A. P., Morales, E. S., & Mays, V. M. (2014). Family culture in mental health help-seeking and utilization in a nationally representative sample of Latinos in the United States: The NLAAS. *American Journal of Orthopsychiatry*, *84*(4), 353. https://doi.org/10.1037/h0099844

Watters, E. (2010). *Crazy like us: The globalization of the American psyche*. Simon and Schuster.

Wechsler, D. (2008). *Wechsler Adult Intelligence Scale-Fourth Edition*. The Psychological Corporation.

Weinstein, E. R., & Jimenez, D. E. (2021). "Gloria a Dios": How spirituality and religiosity can improve healthy cognitive aging interventions for older Latinos. *The American Journal of Geriatric Psychiatry*, *29*(11), 1089–1091. https://doi.org/10.1016/j.jagp.2021.05.012

Weschsler, D. (2014). *Wechsler intelligence scale for children–Fifth Edition (WISC-V)*. Bloomington, MN: Pearson.

Weschsler, D. (1997). *Weschler Adult Intelligence Scale-III*. Psychological Corporation: San Antonio, TX, USA.

Weschler, D., Hernández, A., Aguilar, C., Paradell, E., & Vallar, F. (2015). *Escala de Inteligencia de Wechsler para Niños-V*. Pearson.

Weiss, L. G., Prifitera, A., & Munoz, M. R. (2015). Issues related to intelligence testing with Spanish-speaking clients. In K. F. Geisinger (Ed.), *Psychological testing of Hispanics: Clinical, cultural, and intellectual issues* (pp. 81–107). Washington, DC: American Psychological Association. https://doi.org/10.1037/14668-006

Weiss, L. G., Chen, H., Harris, J. G., Holdnack, J. A., & Saklofske, D. H. (2010). WAIS-IV use in societal context. In Weiss, Saklofske, Coalson, & Raiford (Eds.), *WAIS-IV clinical use and interpretation* (pp. 97–139). Academic Press.

Weschsler, D. (1997). *Weschler Adult Intelligence Scale-III*. Psychological Corporation: San Antonio, TX, USA.

Whitworth, R. H., & McBlaine, D. D. (1993). Comparison of the MMPI and MMPI-2 administered to Anglo-and Hispanic-American university students. *Journal of Personality Assessment*, *61*(1), 19–27.

Whooley, O. (2016). Measuring mental disorders: The failed commensuration project of the DSM5. *Social Science and Medicine*, *166*, 33–40. https://doi.org/10.1016/j.socsci med.2016.08.006

Widaman, K. F., & Reise, S. P. (1997). Exploring the measurement invariance of psychological instruments: Applications in the substance use domain. In K. J. Bryant, M. Windle, & S. G. West (Eds.), *The science of prevention: Methodological advances from alcohol and substance abuse research* (pp. 281–324). Washington, DC: American Psychological Association. https://doi.org/10.1037/10222-009

Wing, J. (1980). Methodological issues in psychiatric case-identification. *Psychological Medicine, 10*(1), 5–10. doi:10.1017/S0033291700039556

Wolff, K. T., Baglivio, M. T., Intravia, J., & Piquero, A. (2015). The protective impact of immigrant concentration on juvenile recidivism: A statewide analysis of youth offenders. *Journal of Criminal Justice, 43*, 522–531. https://doi.org/10.1177/00111 28717739608

Wood, L. C. (2018). Impact of punitive immigration policies, parent–child separation and child detention on the mental health and development of children. *BMJ Paediatrics Open, 18*(1). 1–19. https://doi.org/10.1136/bmjpo-2018-000338

Yearwood, E. L., Crawford, S., Kelly, M., & Moreno, N. (2007). Immigrant youth at risk for disorders of mood: recognizing complex dynamics. *Archives of Psychiatric Nursing, 21*(3), 162–171.

Yoon, E., Chang, C. T., Kim, S., Clawson, A., Cleary, S. E., Hansen, M., . . . Gomes, A. M. (2013). A meta-analysis of acculturation/enculturation and mental health. *Journal of Counseling Psychology, 60*(1), 15.

Zamarripa, M. X., & Lerma, E. (2013). School-based assessment with Latina/o children and adolescents. In L. T. Benuto (Ed.), *Guide to psychological assessment with Hispanics* (pp. 335–349).

For the benefit of digital users, indexed terms that span two pages (e.g., 52–53) may, on occasion, appear on only one of those pages.

Tables are indicated by *t* following the page number